GROWING
Strong

CAMBRIA JOY

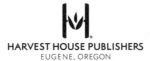

HARVEST HOUSE PUBLISHERS
EUGENE, OREGON

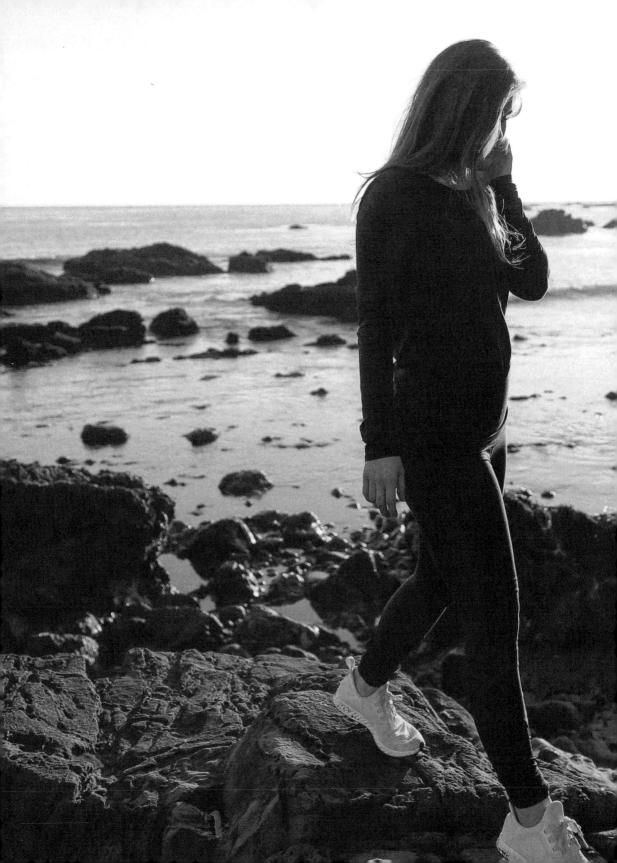

THIS BOOK IS DEDICATED TO ALL OF MY SUBSCRIBERS— YOU ARE MY FRIENDS. THIS BOOK IS FOR YOU. I PRAY YOU MOVE INTO ALL GOD HAS FOR YOU. I LOVE YOU ENDLESSLY! THANK YOU FOR LETTING ME BE A PART OF YOUR LIFE. I'M FOREVER GRATEFUL TO GOD FOR YOU.

CONTENTS

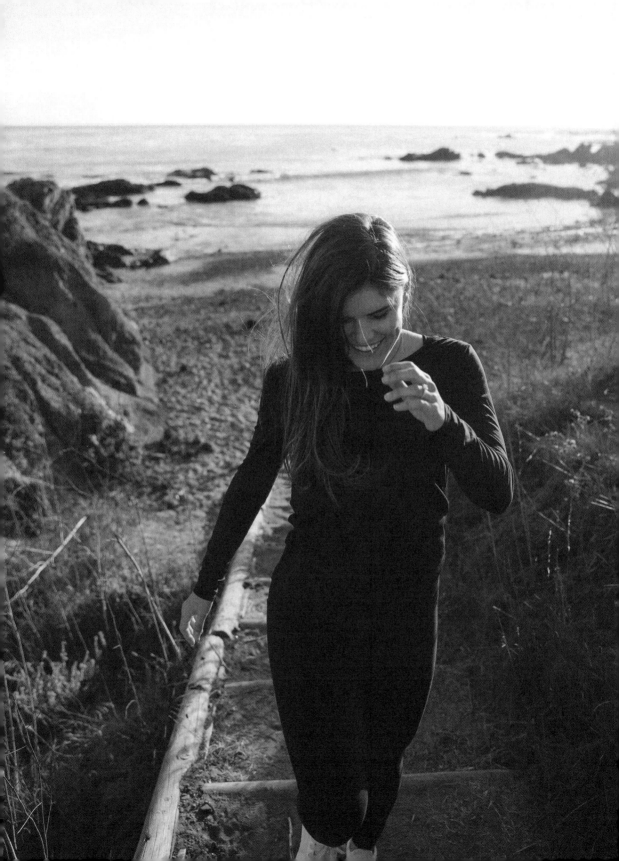

BECOME
You!

THE DESIRE TO BECOME SOMETHING I'M NOT—especially physically— started early in my life. And the more I speak with others, the more certain I am that this is true for many. What else is true? We're all tired of looking in the mirror and criticizing and comparing. We want to know we are loved just as we are. And we're ready to live healthy lives, physically and spiritually.

Maybe you got this book because, like me, you want to be happy and be content with your body and life, but the struggle is real and you lose your way. Some days you aren't even sure what a healthy, content life looks like, am I right?

My friend, this is exactly why I wrote this. We've fixed our eyes so long on the external measures of how and who we are that we believe real beauty is found out there. But God is calling us to turn our eyes away from ourselves, the reflection in the mirror, or the person next to us at the gym. He's inviting us to look to Him for our measure of beauty and worth. First Samuel 16:7 says, "But the Lord said to Samuel, 'Do not look at his appearance or at his physical stature, because I have refused him. For the Lord does not see as man sees; for man looks at the outward appearance, but the Lord looks at the heart.'" When we fix our eyes on Jesus, we are transformed by His truth and can rest in who He says we are.

When you nurture beauty of the spirit, you'll discover a joy that's lasting. This joy, in turn, inspires your pursuit of physical health.

For years I tried to separate my spiritual life and physical life. I prioritized being fit on the outside rather than the inside. And then through spiritual growth and life experiences, I realized that those two things do not have to be separate—in fact, they work in harmony. When you nurture beauty of the spirit, you'll discover a joy that's lasting. This joy, in turn, inspires your pursuit of physical health. I'm excited to come alongside you and encourage this amazing happening in your life.

In case we've never met before, my name is Cambria. I've been working out for almost a decade, and I'm a certified personal trainer through the National Academy of Sports Medicine. Through the ups and downs of trying to live healthy, God has shown me His faithfulness. I had years when my motivation and methods were way off track. Throughout our journey together, I'll honestly share about times of my life that aren't very glamorous. I want to be as open and vulnerable with you here on the page as I am with people I coach in person or online.

If you think everything about my life is picture-perfect, then I'm letting you down. I want to empower you with an understanding of what God has done in my life and will do in your life.

Healthy living opened my eyes to the need for and joy of complete dependence on God. As I became stronger, I longed to have every part of me surrendered to Him. I didn't want to hide the times when I obsessed about my diet and my workouts; instead, I wanted to lean into His love and ask for help.

ENCOURAGEMENT FOR YOUR TRANSFORMATION

I created this journey of encouragement and practical help so you can become fit and whole no matter how you're feeling or which messages from the world happen to be

WE'RE NOT
CREATED TO
perfect our image
BUT TO
reflect His image.

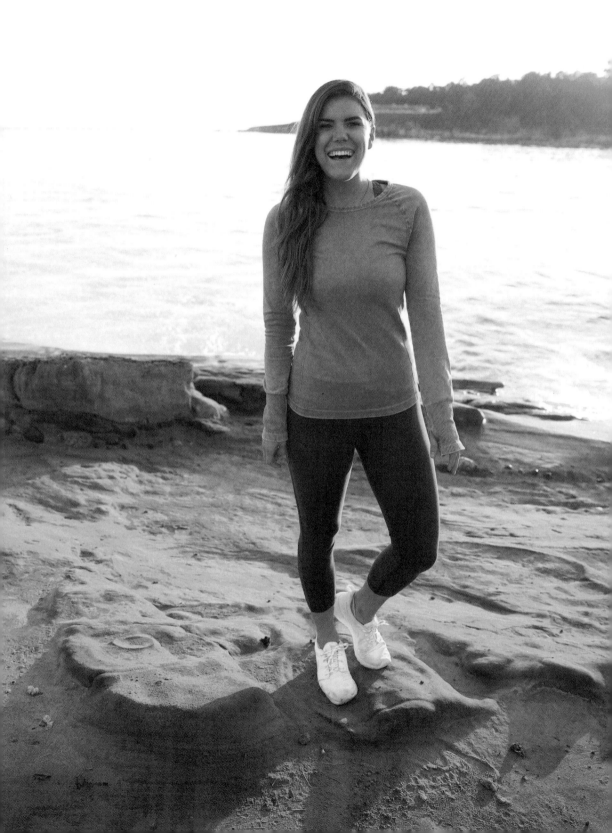

the loudest. Those things change daily, but God's love and His nourishing words are constant. I wrote this to remind you and me that God is the answer to our every need. Let this truth steep in your soul so it can change you. You will be infused and transformed: Like water to tea, you can be changed in the best sort of way. Your life will have more flavor, health, fragrance, and joy.

It doesn't matter how old you are, what shape you're in, or how long you have or haven't been working out; you'll become fit as you nurture your body and soul in healthy ways. I'm eager to share what I've learned. Not because I know it all, but because I understand how tough it can be some days. We'll explore how to **become motivated, become strong, and become transformed**.

If you've joined me online, you've probably heard me say, "We're not created to perfect our image but to reflect His image." When you reflect Jesus through your unique life—not a copy of someone else's life—you'll taste the joy.

FIT FOR JOY—BODY AND SOUL

God wants all of you and all of me. Not to control us, but because He knows that when we focus on Him, we ourselves will thrive. When we know that God loves us perfectly, on the inside and out, we come at this journey from a place of security in our identity in Christ. That's why this journey is about building up the harmony between our physical and spiritual selves. My priority is to provide you with the food, inspiration, and training your body *and* soul need. I'll share from my journey of discovery, and I'll give you plenty of practical support, including...

- easy and nourishing recipes,
- inspirational words, and
- workouts to improve physical strength and health.

I hope you will care for yourself by setting aside time to be encouraged...Pour yourself a hot cup of tea (or make one of the delicious smoothie recipes) and read a portion each day. I wrote it for you.

Imagine a girl who is confident, who knows who she is, who is not afraid of the opinions of others, who stands with her feet firmly planted in the truth, who faces the mirror with bravery in her eyes and a deep love in her heart because she knows who she is in God's eyes. She knows her worth is more precious than rubies and she is fearfully and wonderfully created. She knows that loving God with all her heart, soul, mind, and strength makes her beautiful from the inside out. Her face glows because she is filled with the joy of the Lord. Her lips speak uplifting words to edify herself and others. Her eyes see past her looks and focus on the unseen beauty of a gentle and quiet spirit, which is of infinite worth in God's eyes.

Who's that girl? She is you.

Don't wait for tomorrow when this is an ideal moment to become you. I'll start us off with a prayer. Friend, let's do this together.

From my heart to yours,

Cambria Joy

P.S. To encourage you in your journey, I have created a series of videos featuring each of the workouts in this book. 📹 Turn to page 221 for all the details!

God, teach us to seek You first above all else so that we might please You and be fruitful in all areas of our lives, including healthy living. Show us how to care for ourselves in a way that gives us the energy to serve You and do what You have called us to do. Thank You that we never have to do anything alone, including figuring out how to live healthy. I praise You that we are fearfully and wonderfully made. Help us honor You in everything that we do all the days of our lives. In Jesus's name, amen.

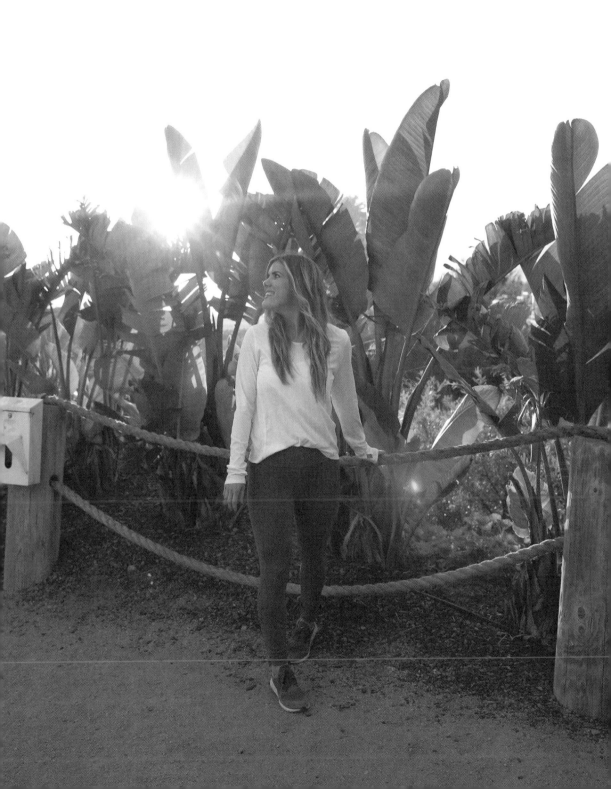

PART
ONE

BECOME
Motivated

I wake up early and roll out of bed with anticipation and joy. I realize that for the first time in a long time, I'm eager for a new day instead of anxious about it.

Within minutes I'm dressed in my workout clothes and have gathered up my hair in a ponytail. I down my preworkout smoothie and walk past the mirror I used to stare at while judging my looks. The only desire I have now is to get to my favorite exercise class.

My drive along the highway showcases breathtaking horizons ahead of me and in my rearview mirror. I say, "Thank You, Lord," for the motivation this beauty gives me to be active first thing.

If I look in the rearview mirror of life, I see scenes from not long ago of me crumpled on my bedroom floor crying, discouraged, broken. My quest for body perfection had driven me to an eating disorder and a soul-deep despair.

I couldn't see a way out. Until God saw a way in: my heart.

Through prayer, feasting on God's Word, and seeking godly counsel, I understood my value and my motivations were reshaped by Jesus.

I pull into the gym's parking lot with a smile on my face. Each day I follow through, I'm more motivated to do it again. And the days that I don't, well, I give myself grace. Unlike the scenes of my past, today's commitment to be fit doesn't come from a spirit of perfection. I'm here because I know nurturing both my body and spirit allows me to more fully live this life for God.

Let's walk forward together with renewed motivation and joy from the Lord.

REFRESH
AND
SATISFY
Your Heart

WHEN I FIRST STARTED MY HEALTHY-LIVING JOURNEY, my goal was to attain happiness by having the perfect body. (In other words, I started an *unhealthy*-living journey.) My motivation was not to become fit, body and soul. Here I thought I was aiming for the ultimate achievement, but I was actually aiming *too* low. Standards that feed and strengthen the spirit are far higher than earthly standards!

If we want to be happy standing in front of the mirror, it has little to do with what we see with our eyes but rather what we know in our hearts. We cannot be good stewards of our bodies if our souls are not aligned with God's heart.

So that's where we're going to start—on the inside. When we align our hearts with God's heart, we can know that we are motivated by what God wants for us. And how do we know God's heart? By knowing His Son Jesus through His Word.

REFRESHED MOTIVATIONS

Our new goal should be to get close to the One who made our souls and bodies. We can't expect inner wholeness to come any other way. Jesus invites us to drink of Him and be fully quenched, and yet our parched souls try to drink from other waters, hoping to be satisfied. There's a story in the Bible in which Jesus speaks to a Samaritan woman at a well. She is there to fetch water in the heat of the day. She is weary and has a troubled life that she and others judge without grace. I can relate, can you?

Chances are, in our unique stories, we have a hardship or struggle that allows us to relate to the weariness and shame of the Samaritan woman.

I have a history of unhealthy motivations and methods for my workouts. I used to binge eat. I based my value on the shape of my body instead of the condition of my heart. My focus on external goals distracted me from the best reason to be fit inside and out: to honor my gifts from God and the person He created me to be. It took me a while to realize that until I pursued transformation from the inside out, I would never be satisfied. Never whole. Always thirsty.

When the Samaritan woman fills her vessel with water, Jesus sees the condition of her heart. He knows that the well water will only satisfy a physical need, yet this woman, like so many of us, has hurts, needs, and hopes that require answers and healing that go beyond the physical. He sees all that comes from her heart and that her motivation is only for physical satisfaction. She is aiming too low. Jesus says to her,

"Whoever drinks of this water will thirst again, but whoever drinks of the water that I shall give him will never thirst. But the water that I shall give him will become in him a fountain of water springing up into everlasting life." JOHN 4:13–14

Each of us is that woman at the well. We're vulnerable and our hearts are aching for someone to notice us. We think our motivations for physical satisfaction are all that matter because that is all we understand until we see our lives through Jesus's eyes and heart. His love and grace change everything. Then we recognize our longing for living water, spiritual refreshment.

JESUS IS CALLING
YOU TO WHAT IS BEST:

*eternal life and
satisfaction in Him.*

Jesus is not saying that if you drink from Him that He will satisfy you by giving you everything you want in this life. No. Jesus is calling you to what is best: eternal life and satisfaction in Him.

Do you believe Jesus can permanently quench your thirst? Is the gospel enough to satisfy you? You will never thirst again when you find your worth in Christ. Your worth then is not found in applause from others. It won't be determined by the accomplishments you reach or even the biggest setbacks you face. I don't like working for things that will ultimately run me dry. How about you?

When you give up the desire for lesser things, you're never losing anything. In fact, you will lose nothing and gain it all.

Ask Jesus to help you be fully satisfied in Him rather than striving for satisfaction. If we pause to remember this each time we seek satisfaction from anything other than Him, we'll be able to reset and refresh our spirits and our motivations.

It is this simple: Jesus Himself satisfies, and if we try to drink from any other waters in hopes of finding what's exclusively found in Him alone, we will thirst again. Satisfaction is a state of the soul, the Bible says in Psalm 107:9: "For He satisfies the longing soul, and fills the hungry soul with goodness." Anytime we set a goal, we need to remember who satisfies. Not *what* satisfies. *Who* satisfies. Jesus Christ satisfies the longing soul.

Do something good for your spiritual and physical heart today. Go on a prayer walk. Memorize a verse to think on while at the gym. Let your soul find rest in Jesus and all of you will be refreshed…including your intentions and heart motivations.

ACTION STEP ——————————————————

Improve digestion today by drinking water 20 minutes before your meal and waiting to drink water at least 20 minutes after your meal. This will keep your stomach acid potent when you are eating and will improve overall digestion!

TOTAL ARM TONER

LEVEL: EASY

TIME: 20 MINUTES WITH REST

ROUTINE: 12 REPS, 4 SETS

I love having strong arms, and this workout is one of my favorites.
It efficiently and effectively targets all the different arm muscles.

▶ TURN TO PAGE 221 TO ACCESS VIDEOS FOR THIS WORKOUT!

BICEP CURL TO OVERHEAD PRESSES

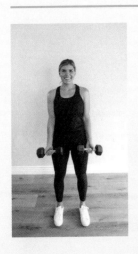 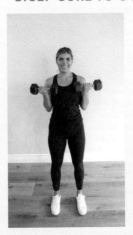 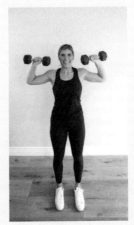 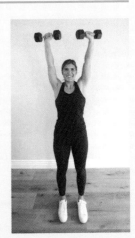

TRICEP KICKBACKS

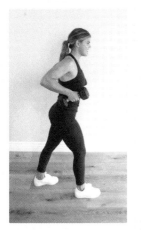 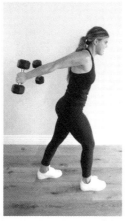 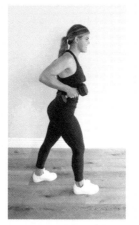 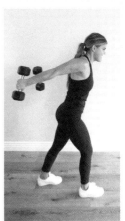

BENT-OVER REVERSE FLYS

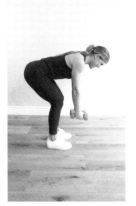 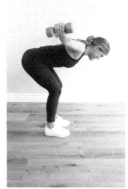 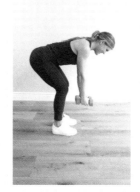 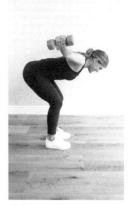

TRICEP OVERHEAD PRESSES

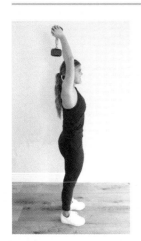 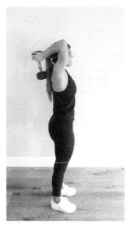 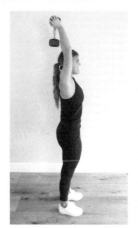 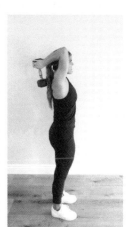

2

TRADE YOUR MAP FOR

God's Plan

I WAS ECSTATIC. AT 15, I WAS STARTING MY FIRST DIET, and I couldn't wait to know exactly what to eat and what to stay away from. I believed that map was all the motivation and direction I would need to become a better, happier version of me.

With great commitment, I stayed true to it...and got nowhere. Actually, I went in the opposite direction of health, myself, and God's truth about me. I was careening along windy paths to an unhealthy relationship with food. I became obsessed with the numbers I used to measure my worth each day: calories, minutes of exercise, pounds on the scale. My body and mind weren't guided by truth and God's love.

The map I chose to follow to discover my lean, ideal self caused me to gain weight. It took me where I didn't want to go and through a lot more harm than help. I was defeated. Running around in circles (sometimes literally) to become something you are not is far from motivating. Each night before sleep, I felt more discouraged than ever.

Have you read Deuteronomy 2:2–3? "And the Lord spoke to me, saying: 'You have skirted this mountain long enough; turn northward.'" That first diet sent me circling the satisfaction mountain for many years, striving for a perfect body. I finally acknowledged that this was more exhausting than heading straight up the mountain. It was time to trust God. I surrendered my life to God and He was faithful. The Lord directed me to stop dieting. Yikes…He found the part of my life I hadn't wanted to give up. Is there anything you are holding this tightly? I wanted control. God knew this, and He knew my distorted perspective couldn't solve my problems. He was the solution.

If you're going in circles, it's time to stop trusting in your map and look to God's plan for you. Do you know what? Colossians 3:3 changed my life: "For you died, and your life is hidden with Christ in God." My identity and hope will not be found in physical gain. Understanding this allowed me to lay down my desire for a perfect body. When I stopped obsessing over my appearance, I eventually stopped bingeing, lost the weight I had gained while bingeing, stopped feeling sick and bloated, let go of perfection, and enjoyed how God designed me…satisfied in Him alone!

GOD'S DIRECTION AND DESIGN

You can trust God's direction in every area of your life. Take Him at His word: "'For I know the plans I have for you,' declares the LORD, 'plans to prosper you and not to harm you, plans to give you hope and a future'" (Jeremiah 29:11 NIV). God has a plan for your body, mind, and spirit to prosper.

God created our bodies with magnificent precision. They're designed to serve our lives so we can serve Him. Within our bodies is a God-designed eating plan. It's called "hungry and full." I know, that sounds too simple, particularly if you've followed severe diet plans like I have. Yet when we listen to our built-in signals, we are guided in the direction of the plans that give us hope. I know this to be true!

Before humans figured out what a calorie was, they weren't counting macros or weighing their food! They ate when they were hungry and stopped when they were full. When we override this, it can lead to unhealthy behavior, like not eating when hungry because we hit the daily calorie limit. Or not eating fruit because it's too high in sugar. Or skimping on avocado because it's too high in fat.

Let's say yes to resting in the finished work of Jesus.

The next time you're hungry, eat until you're satisfied. When you're full, trust your body by saving the next bite for later. Ask God to help you honor how He designed you.

I could regret the day I first carefully mapped out every detail and calorie, but it started me on my journey to trusting God's plan. It was hard to go up the mountain, but we made it together, and metaphorically speaking, the view was worth it. My surrendered heart found truth in the security of God's direction. When your heart finds its worth in Christ alone, you face the question, *Am I going to strive and struggle to live for myself or rest in the finished work of Jesus?*

Jesus doesn't want to compete with anyone or anything in your heart. He created you and knows what's best for you. Throw away your map. Trust that your Creator made you right and His direction is worth following.

ACTION STEP

After your workout, take time to stretch and purposefully pray while you're stretching so that your body and soul can relax.

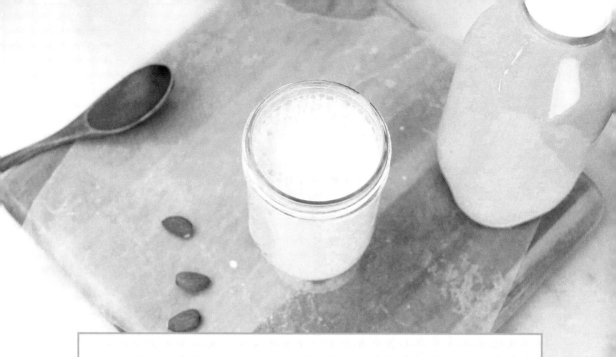

HOMEMADE ALMOND MILK

Homemade almond milk is a total game changer. It's creamy, delicious, free of any additives, and wonderful in lattes. Homemade nut milk is better than store-bought.

PREP TIME: OVERNIGHT **YIELD: 5 CUPS**

---

1 cup almonds (soaked overnight in cool water)
1 tsp. vanilla extract
5 cups filtered water
Pinch of salt

Rinse and drain the almonds. In a high-powered blender, blend the ingredients on high for 1 minute. Strain through a nut milk bag. Shake before each use.

3

GAIN
momentum

"HOW DO I GET AND *STAY* MOTIVATED?"

I get this question more than any other from my online community. And believe me, I need to be reminded of the answer. Particularly after a low-energy week or a season of life that interrupts my routines. I'm living in such a time right now, as a matter of fact.

The key to staying motivated is to be sure that everything important—intentions, motives, focus, source of validation—is in its rightful place and that you are going the right direction.

How can you be sure? It happens when you put God in His rightful place in your life and heart: first. Everything and everyone else is second. When you fill yourself up with more of Him, you will find more freedom and joy than you could experience any other way. The verse John 3:30 declares, "He must increase, but I must decrease."

God will help you reshape the motives of your heart so they're stronger and fueled by His purposes. How do I know that? Because He's done that for me. He's gotten me off my own course and onto His. He's prepared the path before me and gone every step of the way with me. As I fix my mind on Him, He changes my heart to beat in sync with His. My steps align with His, and I have confidence because He is my focus and my value comes from Him alone.

YOUR FOCUS AND YOUR FOUNDATION

The big life shift to place God as our priority doesn't lessen the importance of the other valued aspects of our journeys, such as family, friends, love, church, community, purpose, and physical and spiritual health. Those priorities, when put into perspective, are more enjoyable to nurture and our investments in them bear more fruit. Why? Because those areas of focus are no longer responsible for your contentment, self-worth, or your direction in life. You don't look to them for affirmation that you matter. You have a fixed focal point: Jesus.

Now you can volunteer for a community organization without needing the validation of being noticed for it. You can be a friend to the person at work whom you would have wanted to compete with if your sense of worth came only from your job. Tending to your spiritual health with prayer and reading the Bible become ways to nurture your focus on Jesus, and as a result, you become a person who lives out the truths you're reading and the purpose you are called to fulfill. Jesus becomes your focal point and your foundation.

When my priority was not God, my motivations were always changing! One month, I was motivated to try to look good for someone, and the next month, my motivation to be fit was *to* fit into a pair of jeans. The month after, my motivation was to achieve a certain number of workout reps to secretly compete with a girl at the gym. Then when God had His rightful place as number one in my heart, I was motivated to work out and eat to strengthen and fuel my body because God created it. I filled my body with nutrients rather than denying it essential calories. I took pleasure in seeing my muscles become strong and defined not because they fit anyone's standard but because my actions were aligning with what God created my body to do: grow and flourish.

I encourage you to make this shift. Put God in His rightful place in your heart and the other matters will line up. When your identity is secure as God's daughter, you no longer feel pressure to chase changing worldly motivations or goals. You have a calling to become *you* and to honor God along the way. There's no stopping your momentum when your confidence comes from knowing who you are in Christ.

ACTION STEP

Choose a special journal for this journey. Or even two—one for your fitness, food, and feelings and one to be your prayer journal. Whatever serves your style best!

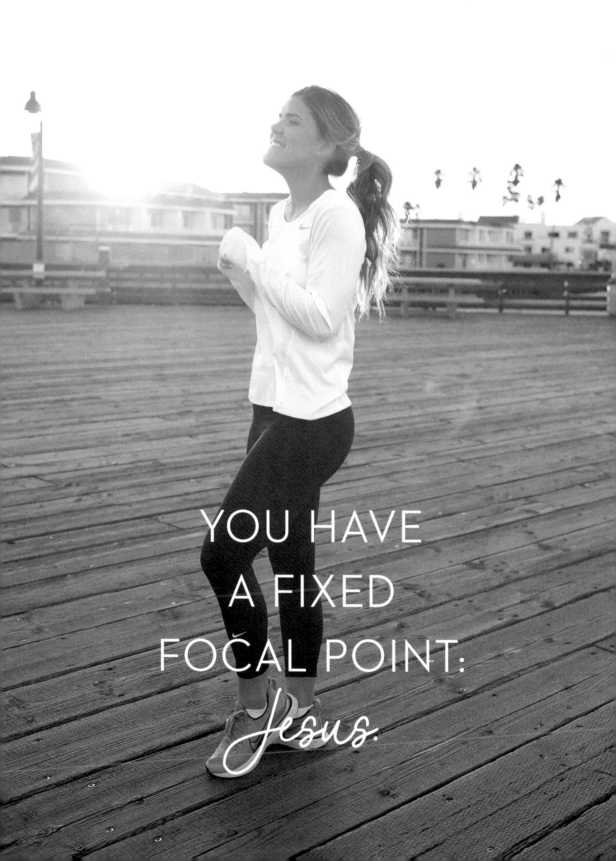

YOU HAVE
A FIXED
FOCAL POINT:
Jesus.

4

STOP DIGGING FOR FALSE *Treasure*

THIN SEEMS TO ALWAYS BE IN. I used to believe that being thinner would make me happier. That being thinner would make people like me more. That being thinner would make me like me more. In fact, I believed those lies for such a long time, the goal of being thinner became the dearest hope in my deceived heart. This false hope consumed me and took my mind off Jesus. James 1:14 says, "But each one is tempted when he is drawn away by his own desires and enticed." While it makes my heart ache to write these words now, they are true: I desired more than anything to be skinny.

My heart's treasure was to attain skinny, but that's fool's gold. False treasure may look pretty, but ultimately it holds no value or worth. It's just nice to look at. That's why we need to be careful when we place our desires above God's truth. Don't let the desires of your heart deceive you into settling for fool's gold.

We try to find treasure in what we think is good, but that search leads us on a scavenger hunt that has no end, no reward, and no life. Some people follow distractions until their time runs out. The Bible says in Proverbs 14:12 that "there is a way that seems right to a man, but its end is the way of death." That's what happened when I believed the lie that my greatest treasure would be found when I finally attained my perfect body. I ran after the rainbow of "skinny = happiness" for years.

ETERNAL-TREASURE HUNT

So where is the real treasure found? It's found in Jesus Christ. So how do we protect our minds from falling victim to the fascination of fool's gold and our hearts from chasing after our own desires? Romans 13:14 says to "put on the Lord Jesus Christ, and make no provision for the flesh, to fulfill its lusts." Put on the Lord and put away the shovel. Stop digging for something that will never satisfy the soul.

Do you want a truth-treasure map? Here it is:

- Choose today to believe His Truth instead.
- Confess to Him the things you have chased after instead of Him.
- Decide you will no longer feed any desire that wants to be first in your heart.
- Refuse to feed thoughts that pull you away from truth.
- Put on Jesus, and you will discover He is the treasure you've been looking for.

Save yourself the heartache and lost time. Don't keep digging for a treasure that will have no eternal value. Those objects that sparkle and capture our attention are the treasures that end up rusting and falling apart.

You and I don't want the debris—we want the victory.

ACTION STEP ————————————————

Build your habit of healthy cooking. Try one of the recipes in this book today and tag me on Instagram @cambriajoy. I can't wait to see your re-creations!

ALL-BODY TONER

LEVEL: **MODERATE**

TIME: **27–36 MINUTES WITH REST**

ROUTINE: **DO EACH EXERCISE FOR 1 MINUTE, 4 SETS**

*Don't let being short on time keep you from breaking a sweat.
Rest up to 1 minute between each movement. This simple but effective
workout will improve your cardio-vascular health and muscle tone.*

▶ TURN TO PAGE 221 TO ACCESS VIDEOS FOR THIS WORKOUT!

JUMPING ROPE

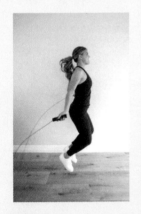
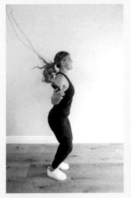
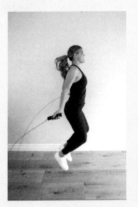
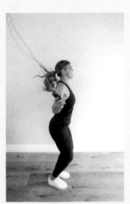

PLANK

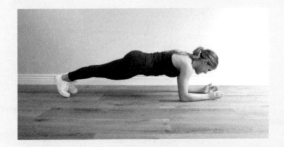
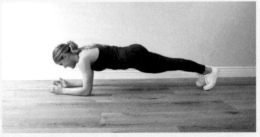

SQUATS

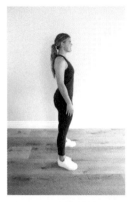 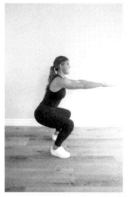 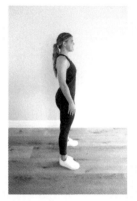 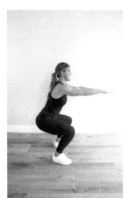

JUMP SQUATS

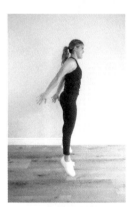 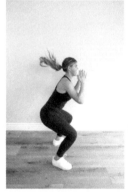 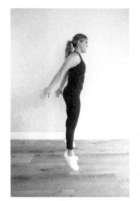 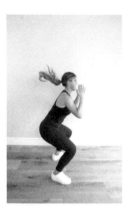

JUMPING JACKS

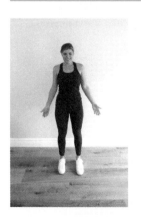 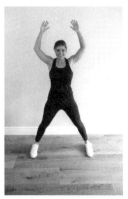 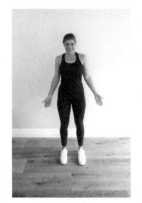 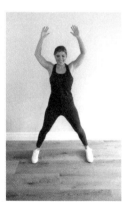

5

IMPROVE YOUR *Playlist*

YOU HAVE AN OPPORTUNITY FOR CHANGE.

Not just a physical change but a mental one. I used to think I was motivating myself by being self-critical. While I worked out, my mind taunted me: *Wow, this is already so hard, and I'm out of breath. Why has it taken me so long to get back into working out? Ugh! I'm so out of shape. I better push through this or I'm never going to be happy with my body!*

Nothing squashes motivation more than a lousy playlist blaring in your ears.

If you also have a familiar shame soundtrack running on repeat, I have great news: You can clean out the unwanted extended play of negative songs, and instead add in and focus on lyrics of love, hope, and faith.

Ephesians 4:29 says, "Let no corrupt word proceed out of your mouth, but what is good for necessary edification, that it may impart grace to the hearers." What if we applied this verse to ourselves and our minds? We'd be working out and living to a different tune. A mix with grace and hope sounds like this: "Wow, this is already so hard. But that's okay! I'm going to push through this because I'm strong. I can do this. I got this. I'm taking care of the body that God gave me, and I'm proud of myself for showing up today."

If the voice in your head isn't lovely
or kind, don't listen to it.

SWITCH CHANNELS

You'll love listening to God. He is not the author and speaker of condemnation or confusion. He is merciful, gracious, slow to anger, and abounding in mercy (Psalm 103:8). Your path of transformation physically and spiritually becomes one of joy when you learn to discern which words are His and listen accordingly. When you're victorious, listen for the voice that builds you up. When you struggle, you'll hear His correction and wisdom.

Don't entertain thoughts that have no business being there in the first place. If the voice in your head isn't lovely or kind, don't listen to it. Tune out the loud bullying voices and listen for God's loving whispers. Ask God to help you tell the difference between His voice of loving conviction and the enemy's voice of condemnation. Ask Him to help you retrain your mind to only listen to the thoughts that come from Him. Which come from Him? If you're unsure about the source of the voice in your head, see if it lines up with the character of God. Is it merciful, gracious, slow to anger, and full of mercy? Learn to listen to the voice of love and you'll discover that other thoughts have no room in your head or heart.

You'll know the Holy Spirit's voice because it leads you to the cross, and you'll know the enemy's voice because it drives you away from the cross. When we stop listening to lies, we'll hear the melodies of grace and knowledge from God.

NO MORE LIE-TUNES

Did you know that everything you do flows from your heart? That's what Proverbs 4:23 says. If we protect, or clean up, our minds and hearts, everything in our life will be graced by that decision. How can we really do this? Let's look at this verse for guidance: "Casting down arguments and every high thing that exalts itself against

> ## You'll know the Holy Spirit's voice because it leads you to the cross.

the knowledge of God, bringing every thought into captivity to the obedience of Christ" (2 Corinthians 10:5). Anything that tries to exalt itself against the knowledge of God is a lie, and we are to bring that thought into the light of truth, where those lies can't hide.

Next time you're at the gym crushing your workout but crushing thoughts are threatening to take over, edify your heart and mind. What does that mean? It means to instruct or improve. Edify your thoughts by making them obedient to Christ. Don't give that chorus of lies a chance to amp up the downbeat. Bring those thoughts to Jesus. Add to your spiritual, mental soundtrack with sound wisdom from God's Word and His heart.

Do this in a practical way too, friend. Create a playlist of Christian songs that motivate you physically and spiritually.

ACTION STEP

Practice moderation today. No suggestion for this one—apply this principle to your life in whatever way it fits you.

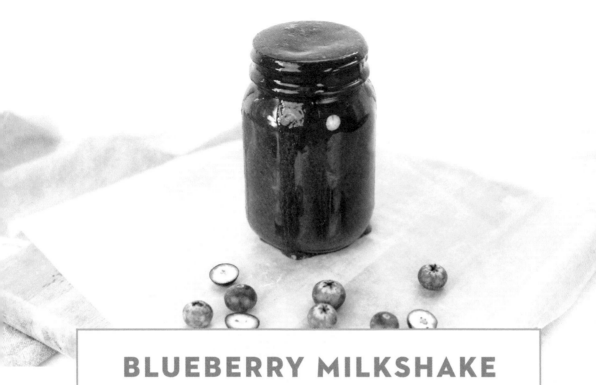

BLUEBERRY MILKSHAKE

*Ah, milkshakes are refreshing. Enhance a classic with vitamins
and almond milk. I recommend freezing your fruit for smoothies
to create a thick and creamy texture.*

PREP TIME: **5 MINUTES**   YIELD: **1 SERVING**

---

³/₄ cup frozen blueberries
1 frozen banana
1 cup almond milk
1 small handful spinach
1 tsp. honey

Blend the ingredients and enjoy for a delicious and
antioxidant-packed berry breakfast or snack.

6

TAKE
One Step

WORKING OUT IS HARD, BUT DO YOU KNOW WHAT'S HARDER?
Actually getting motivated to work out. Holding the last ten seconds of a plank is challenging, but it's more challenging to get yourself to the gym in the first place! It's not that our bodies won't do a burpee, run a mile, or hold a squat. It's that our mind stops us before we get that far. What's the problem here? Well, it's a reality both of us have probably faced: Motivation isn't a physical battle but a mental one.

When we see people who consistently work out, we might assume they're just born with motivation. But the secret sauce of their success is their ability to be unafraid of performing poorly. If you want to change your life, you must be able to tolerate imperfection—dare I say, welcome it—and see it as a teacher and even a friend.

I believe we're all on track toward something. For myself and for many of the people I interact with as a part of my vocation, that track is often perfectionism.

Have you ever felt...

- discouraged after striving for fitness and not seeing results,
- disappointed because you ate a brownie at night after "eating healthy" all day,

- defeated after deciding your body isn't as beautiful as hers, or
- derailed because you missed a workout after trying your best all week?

When we put ourselves on these restrictive tracks, our motivation deflates as soon as we've violated one of our internal laws (a.k.a. lies) of "staying on track." We buy into the lie that someone else is doing it better, so we might as well give up. We buy into the lie that if we don't do it perfectly or we don't see immediate results, we might as well not do it at all.

We act in accordance with how we think, so if you think you've fallen off track, you will start living that way. You live in a perpetual state of unmotivation because you believe you are just plain unmotivated. The good news is that's not true! Get on track with your perfect God rather than for perfection. The lies will fall away and no longer have power over you and your actions.

EMBRACE GRACE

In God, you are mentally strong. I want to scream it from the rooftops: You are capable of reaching goals and chasing God's dream for you! You are not unmotivated; you just need to be reminded of the truth of who you are and the truth about how to be healthy. It really does set you free. The secret, my friend, is to kiss perfection goodbye and embrace grace. Here's how:

- When you work out for ten minutes, believe that it *is* enough.
- Enjoy your dessert. (That's healthy for the soul! And healthy in general—stay away from restrictive eating.)
- Move forward by taking imperfect steps.
- Get up after you fall and keep going.
- Quit carrying lies so you can be light and free in God's truth.

A frequent obstacle to a person's progression and persistence along God's track is being overwhelmed by too many lies, too many self-imposed expectations. Discouragement can set in and you become stuck. Motivation comes when you toss the lies and you keep going. One. Step. At. A. Time.

Get on track with your perfect God rather than for perfection.

Become motivated, stay on track, eat healthy, work out, and care for your body by following God's lead and one of these simple one-step approaches anytime you feel unmotivated:

- Set aside those feelings (lies) and put on your exercise clothes, or
- head to the gym (or your at-home gym), or
- turn on your music, or
- do your warm-up or even just one jumping jack. You're free to decide if you will keep going or head home.

This might seem too simple. My advice? Start looking for simple solutions in your life. Simple works! Set aside the feelings of unmotivation and take one step with God.

ACTION STEP

Pray and specifically ask God to help you take one step toward your health goals today.

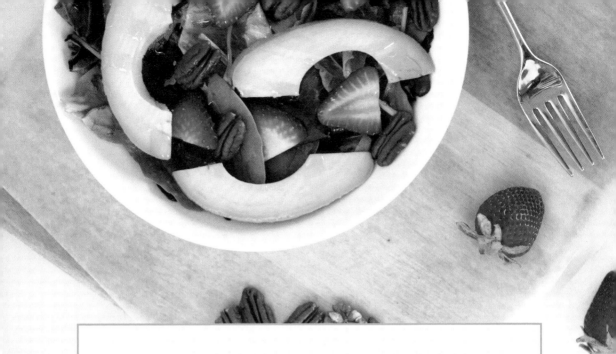

STRAWBERRY-PECAN FIELD SALAD

This tasty field salad is refreshing and packed with micronutrients and healthy fats that are sure to leave your skin glowing. It's my go-to recipe for potlucks.

PREP TIME: **10 MINUTES**   YIELD: **1 SERVING**

Strawberries
Toasted pecans
Avocado
Mixed greens

1 T. coconut aminos
1 T. avocado oil
1 tsp. apple cider vinegar

Chop the strawberries, pecans, and avocado, and top the mixed greens with them. Combine the liquid ingredients and drizzle them over the salad. Serve right away.

7

DON'T
Drift

MY HUSBAND, BO, LOVES TO SURF, and I love watching him. After more than 20 minutes of "the search"—watching the waves—Bo chooses the best spot to run out and catch them. I unfold my floral-print beach chair and plant it down into the sand right in front of the spot where he chooses to surf. I dig my toes into the warm sand and pull out my phone to capture the perfect video angle of him gliding over the water on his surfboard.

Yet something interesting happens every time I have my perfect spot and my precise video location. Slowly, but surely, I lose my front-row seat to his surfing session. Why? Bo unknowingly drifts down the beach because the current is pulling him away from where he intended to go.

A surfer doesn't drift down the entire beach after surfing one wave. It happens gradually as wave after wave causes shifts. If Bo keeps his eyes on me as his anchor point, then after every wave, he can paddle back over a few yards to his particular spot. If he's not referencing the object that is constant (a.k.a. me), he will drift.

My false anchor caused me to drift away
from truth with each wave of uncertainty.

Sometimes we drift off in our life, unaware that we're being swept out to sea. My anchor in my healthy lifestyle used to be looking good. I fixed my eyes on my appearance. Over time, my false anchor caused me to drift away from truth with each wave of uncertainty. Sometimes I drifted because I compared my body to an image online or because I was disappointed that I didn't feel better after reaching a goal. I was lost in the sea of lies and was drowning in discouragement.

ANCHOR OF TRUTH

If we don't want to drift, we must have an anchor that works.

What makes an anchor work? Its weight. What makes a spiritual anchor work? The weight of truth. When we make God's truth our anchor, we stop drifting as we make decisions and set our intentions.

Let the truth that nothing will satisfy your longing except for God anchor you on the days when comparison rushes in. Let it ground you when discouragement tries to take you out. Let it secure you when you take a day of rest and guilt starts to rush over you. You'll discover that the things that used to rock and sway you no longer have that power. You'll find a peace that comes not from a perfect outward appearance but from a secure identity in Christ.

Waves of discouragement and comparison will hit all of us, but they don't have to pull us away from our intended goal. The difference now is that when the tide rises, your anchor is secure, your anchor is constant—your anchor is God's truth.

ACTION STEP

Drink one glass of water before your morning coffee.

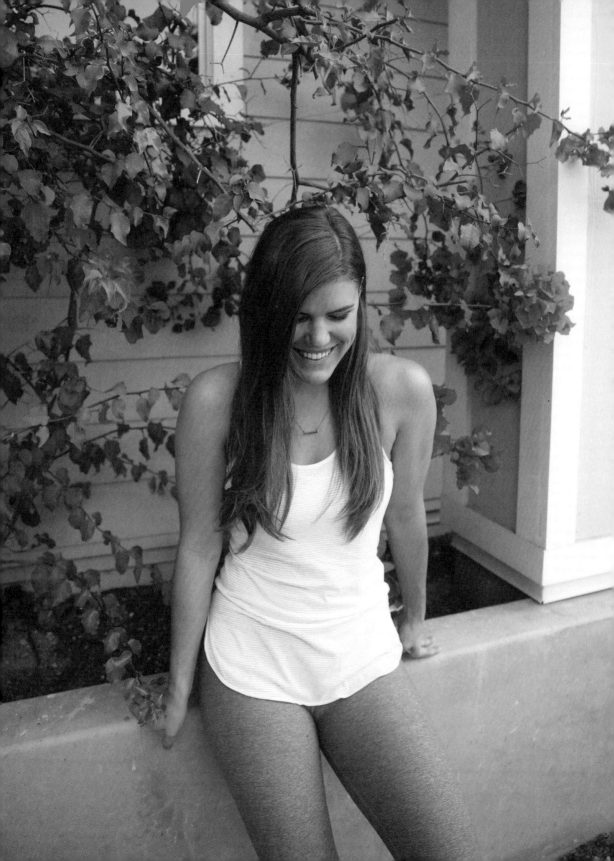

KNOW YOUR VALUE

Spend time feeding your spirit today with words from God reminding you of your great value. Don't ever doubt that you are a treasured woman.

Blessed is she who has believed that the Lord would fulfill his promises to her!

LUKE 1:45 NIV

The Lord said to Samuel, "Do not look on his appearance or on the height of his stature, because I have rejected him. For the Lord sees not as man sees: man looks on the outward appearance, but the Lord looks on the heart."

1 SAMUEL 16:7 ESV

God is within her, she will not fall; God will help her at break of day.

PSALM 46:5 NIV

You were bought with a price.

1 CORINTHIANS 6:20 ESV

If anyone is in Christ, he is a new creation; old things have passed away; behold, all things have become new.

2 CORINTHIANS 5:17

Lord, You know me, love me, and renew me as I journey along the path You have for me. Guide me every step of the way on this journey, and let patience have its perfect work in me so that I stay motivated and grateful. I'm so grateful that You love me and that my value comes from You. In Jesus's name, amen.

8

SHAKE
It Off

GUILT IS A WEIGHT THAT SLOWS US DOWN IF we're not careful to shake it off so that we can run freely.

Have you gotten frustrated with yourself on your fitness journey? Don't condemn yourself for not making progress when you're carrying a load you're not meant to carry! Grace will take you a lot further than guilt. Guilt weighs you down and adds lies and frustrations to your load. It says you can't go on and aren't worthy to. Grace says to take the next step even after you've fallen a thousand times.

Grace will carry you, and guilt will kick you when you're down.

It's time to shake off the weight of guilt and embrace the lightness of grace. John 1:14 says that Jesus is full of grace and truth. And that, my friend, is how we will move forward—by God's grace and with His truth.

Lamentations 3:22–23 (ESV) tells us, "The steadfast love of the LORD never ceases; his mercies never come to an end; they are new every morning." My life changed when I started receiving those new mercies rather than accepting my negative attitude of defeat. I know you don't want to merely survive and face constant guilt and condemnation. You want to be an overcomer who walks in grace and freedom.

NEW MERCIES

Are you living each day with new mercies? Do you wake up every day breathing in a fresh start? Here are some ways you can look at a failing and shake it off and remain on the path designed for you with complete hope and renewed energy.

1. Lean into God's strength. We know that we need something greater than ourselves to get us out of this, and it's only found in the power of God. His power lives in you, and He will enable you to rise above your limits and set you back on your feet again. We can be liberated from our slavery to shame, perfection, and guilt and get back on track when we ask God to help us. God is "able to do exceedingly abundantly above all that we ask or think, according to the power that works in us" (Ephesians 3:20).

2. Forgive yourself. Remember? Embrace that grace. There's no need to wallow in yesterday's mistakes. There is a better way to live! You've got to dust yourself off every single day.

3. View mistakes in a new light. Your failure will not derail you from your purpose when you trust God's way. You're a human and you're going to mess up! Remember the way of grace. Look at your setback as your comeback moment. Don't lie on your back for two days because you've tripped over a pebble. Get up and dust yourself off. Remind yourself that you are created on purpose, for a purpose.

4. Don't dwell on your past. Your past does not need to have a grip on you when you walk in the forgiveness of today. God's mercies are new every single morning. You won't be able to move forward today if you are constantly thinking about yesterday and your missteps.

5. Renew your mind in the truth. When discouragement makes an appearance, or to keep lies from becoming your foundation, refresh and renew your mind with God's Word. Read God's promises and cling to them. The Bible says to take every thought captive and make it obedient to Christ (2 Corinthians 10:5). If we are transformed by the renewing of our minds, then we must pay careful attention to what we are thinking about. Instead of beating yourself up for making a mistake, remember that there's fresh grace for each moment.

6. Know who you are and whose you are. You're an overcomer because you are God's child and He has a plan for good for your life. He will not leave you to yourself, He will help you, He is with you, and you are loved, forgiven, and restored.

Whatever discouragement or setback you are experiencing right now, shake it off.

ACTION STEP

Make your water more fun by adding strawberries, cucumber, and mint—one of my favorite combinations!

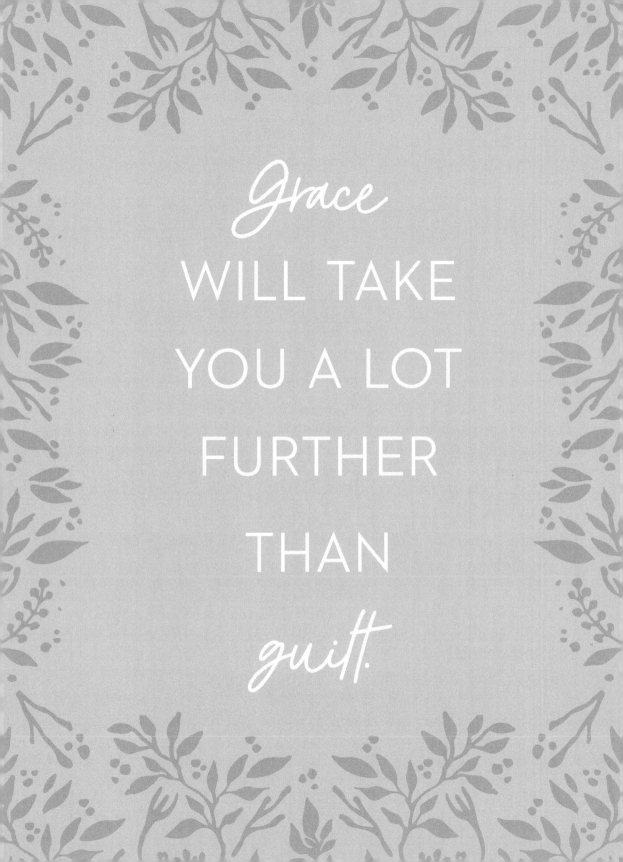

Grace
WILL TAKE
YOU A LOT
FURTHER
THAN
guilt.

9

FACE

Forward

IF WE WANT TO MOVE FORWARD, then we've got to face forward. Where we're looking determines where we're going. If we want to become strong, our attention needs to be on what God has for us right now.

All my mistakes led me to realize that I can't find inner contentment by chasing outward perfection. I was chasing things that don't exist. A perfect body doesn't exist, and a soul-deep happiness apart from God doesn't exist. Whatever mistakes you've made in your past, whether they happened one year ago or one minute ago, shouldn't be your focus. They have been a crucial part of the journey, but they aren't your whole story. The rest of your story lies up ahead.

You and I are here because of grace. God picks us up when we've fallen. He redirects our gaze to be set on Him. When your spirit is downcast, look up and face forward because God has something beautiful on the horizon. God hasn't brought us this far for nothing.

Therefore, since we are surrounded by so great a cloud of witnesses, let us also lay aside every weight, and sin which clings so closely, and let us run with endurance the race that is set before us, looking to Jesus, the founder and perfecter of our faith, who for the joy that was set before him endured the cross, despising the shame, and is seated at the right hand of the throne of God. HEBREWS 12:1-2 ESV

God hasn't brought us this far for nothing.

How did Jesus endure the weight of the world? He was looking ahead to the joy. Ahead was the resurrection, the joy of obedience on the cross, and the joy of being at the right hand of the throne of God.

JOY IS AHEAD

Get your eyes off your mistakes and on your future. Stop trying to fix yesterday and start living in the beauty of today by remembering that joy is in front of you right now. In our lifetimes, we can look forward to the plans God has for us. And ahead of that is eternity. There is great joy for you and me.

Are you ready for a fresh start and to move into all God has for you?

If you are, then don't give up, look up. God wants to get you on course. If you are hanging your head out of shame for past mistakes, hold on to this hope: "But You, O Lord, are a shield for me, my glory and the One who lifts up my head" (Psalm 3:3). God is our shield against the lies that tell us we'll never be able to move forward, and when our eyes can't seem to find their way up, God lifts our heads and shows us the view of hope. Don't look back and feel discouraged, face forward and be encouraged because there is a whole lot of joy to be experienced! You want to be a witness to all that God has for you today.

When you face forward, focus on today rather than jumping ahead to thoughts or concerns about tomorrow. God tells us not to worry about tomorrow. The only thing we need to think on for the next day is that God has gone before us and prepared the way. Rest in that, friend. God works all things together for good because that's His promise. Face forward and put your hope in the joy of this moment.

ACTION STEP

Try incorporating gut-healthy foods into your diet today such as sauerkraut, coconut oil, bone broth, apple cider vinegar, or yogurt.

I GOT YOUR BACK!

LEVEL: EASY

TIME: 25 MINUTES WITH REST

ROUTINE: 12 REPS, 4 SETS

This workout is perfect for strengthening your back. Rest as needed, however, I recommend little to no rest between movements. Rest up to 1 minute between sets.

Modify: Start with no weights and then progress to 1-pound, 3-pound, and 5-pound weights in time.

▶ TURN TO PAGE 221 TO ACCESS VIDEOS FOR THIS WORKOUT!

SUPERMANS

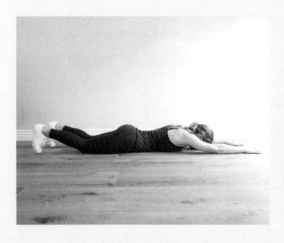 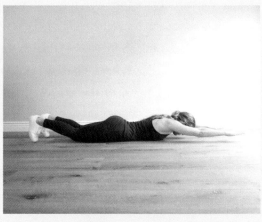

BENT-OVER ROWS

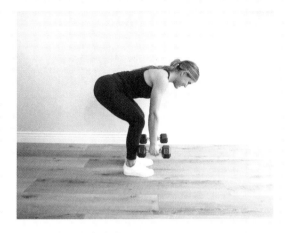 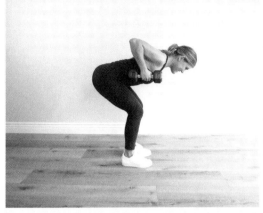

BENT-OVER REVERSE FLYS

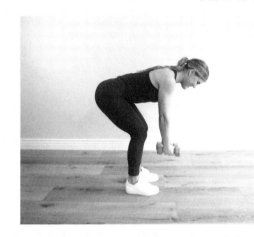 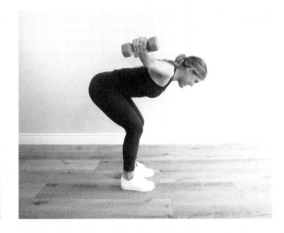

OVERHEAD PRESSES

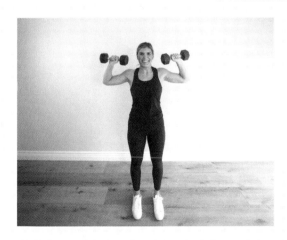 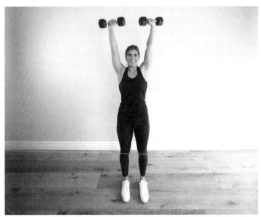

10

STAY IN
Your Lane

HAVE YOU BEEN THERE, on the sidelines peering at what someone else is accomplishing in their personal journey while you're frustrated with your own?

I've peeked over at the other girl's treadmill before. I've scrolled through endless feeds and felt jealous, like I'm not doing enough and I'll never be enough. Someone else seems to always be doing more or at least better. She is more successful. I've definitely drifted out of my own lane and onto the sidelines to watch others run their races.

Comparison potentially makes us...

- feel like we need to do more,
- forget who we are,
- want to give up.

Do you find yourself discouraged, jealous, envious, hopeless, worried, resentful, or full of self-pity after you've compared your life to someone else's? Do you feel

> ## If something costs you your peace,
> ## then it's too expensive.

powerless to quit resorting to comparison once and for all? We can overcome what wants to overcome us with prayer and through the truth of God's Word.

You can surrender comparison when you realize that your life is secure in God and He is leading you on the best path for your life.

THE COST OF COMPARISON

We've all heard that if something costs you your peace, then it's too expensive. Comparison left unremoved from your heart can grow into envy. Envy comes at too high of a cost because look at the end result: Proverbs 14:30 says, "A sound heart is life to the body, but envy is rottenness to the bones."

I've found that the times I've been the most envious are the times that I've been insecure. God wants you to be secure in Him. Comparison left unchecked can grow roots of bitterness. Hebrews 12:15 says, "[Look] carefully lest anyone fall short of the grace of God; lest any root of bitterness springing up cause trouble, and by this many become defiled."

Who wants rottenness when we're aiming to be healthy and joyful in God? Who wants to trip and tumble over roots of bitterness while running the path, living the life, and nourishing the body God gives us?

On the other hand, if we're sowing God's truth into our hearts, we will be strong and secure in God's love for us. Remember the story of the woman at the well we explored earlier? Jesus wanted her to have the living water. He wants us to be satisfied in Him alone and secure in who He made us to be. That is what will refresh our journey and give us encouragement, motivation, and the ability to run our race.

I caught myself comparing just the other night, and the first thing I did was pray. I prayed that God would fill me up with His love and that I would stay true to His specific purpose and plan for my life.

We can lay comparison down when we follow the truth of who we are in Christ. The truth that you don't need to do more. The truth that you don't need to try harder.

Who you are in Him is enough.

ACTION STEP

Take 30 minutes today to do some meal prep: Chop up veggies, make some granola, or prepack smoothies for an even more convenient snack.

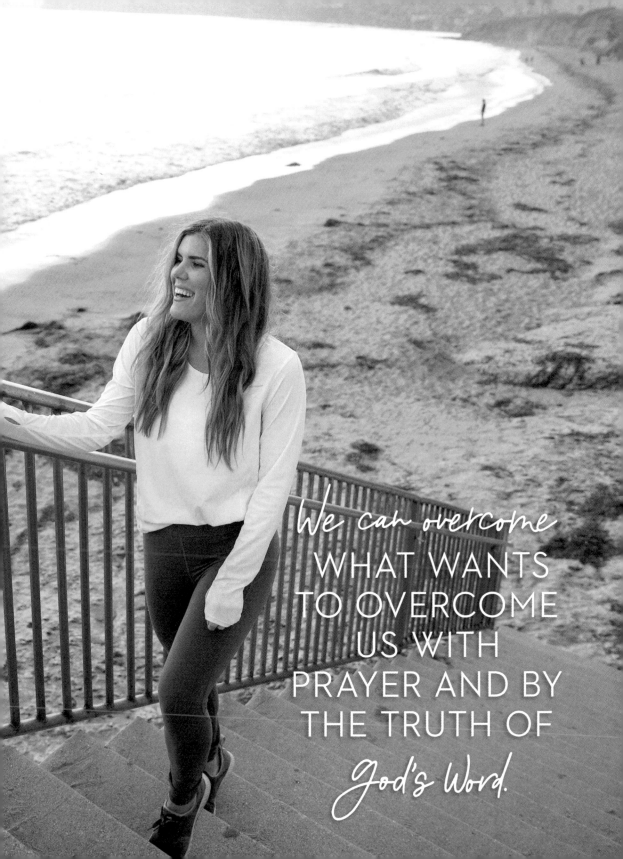

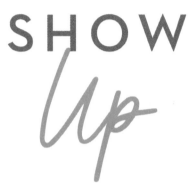

SHOW *Up*

IN HIGH SCHOOL, I TRIED OUT FOR WATER POLO. To make the team, I had to survive what they called "hell week." It was definitely harsh. I had to wake up at 4:30 a.m. to be at school on time to swim a crazy number of laps and perform endless rounds of treading water. If we didn't show up each day, then we would be cut from the team.

Well, 15-year-old Cambria showed up. I wasn't good. In fact, I was probably the worst on the team. Wait, let's be honest—I *was* the worst on the team. My weak point was that I could barely tread water and my strong point was swallowing water.

I was so bad at treading water that one of the older girls on the team was assigned to teach me how to "eggbeater," which is the treading technique used by water polo players. I was the only one who needed extra help. How humiliating. As much as the patient upperclassmen tried to teach me, I could not coordinate my legs and arm movements. Day after day, I tried, and I failed. However, the end of that treacherous week finally arrived…and so did I.

I made it through the week. I couldn't believe it. Did I successfully learn how to eggbeater? No. But did I show up every day and get through practice? Yes, by the grace of God, I did.

Whatever you do, don't give up.

Here's the key: I wouldn't get cut if I didn't know how to eggbeater. I would get cut if I didn't show up. It's one thing to not be good at what you're doing; it's another thing to not try at all.

WHAT OR WHO WILL YOU SHOW UP FOR?

It's not how good you are at something that matters; it's your willingness to show up and do it. This is true when applying for a job, auditioning for a play, or reaching out in friendship at the risk of rejection, it is certainly true in our pursuit of living healthy.

Whether you're new to working out or trying to eat in a way that makes your body feel good, you've got to show up every single day. Don't be afraid to fail. Don't let your thoughts churn with anxiety, wondering "what if" you don't succeed in the way you want. Because guess what? Sometimes achievement looks different from what you imagined. Or a victory comes later than hoped: I eventually learned how to eggbeater. It took me weeks, but I did it.

As you set forth to try something, ask God to help you. He will help your body, mind, and spirit in ways you can't imagine or plan. Turn to the encouragement of Galatians 6:9 (NIV): "Let us not become weary in doing good, for at the proper time we will reap a harvest if we do not give up." Whatever you do, don't give up. No matter how long it takes, be encouraged, knowing that you're going to eventually reap what you sow. And guess what? You will reap right when the harvest is right.

God's timing is perfect, and the patience and endurance you learn along the way are just as sweet as the harvest itself.

ACTION STEP ——————————————————————

Time for a little TLC. Take an Epsom salt bath today and have a nice long foam roll and stretch.

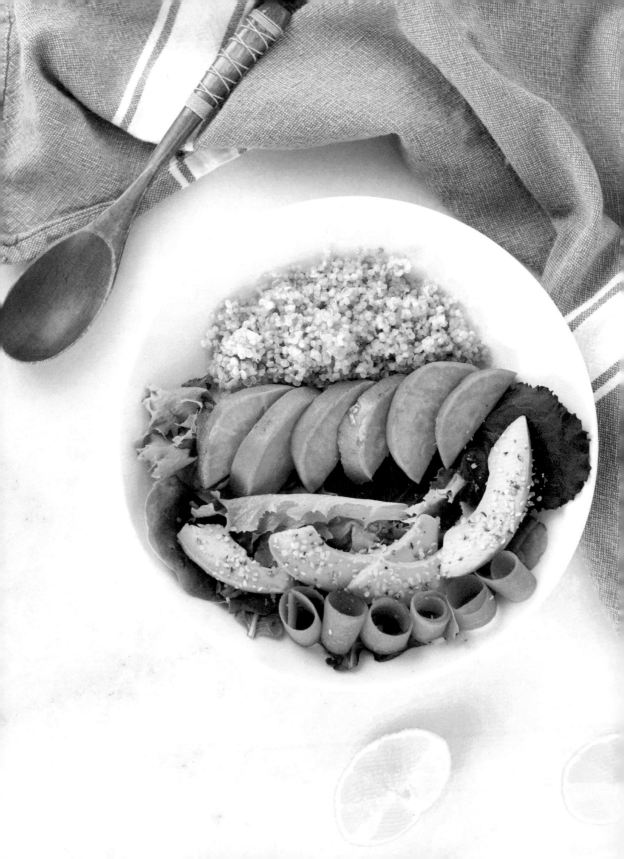

SIMPLE NOURISH BOWL

The classic nourish bowl—customizable, healthy, and most importantly, delicious. This simple dinner is perfect to whip up on a whim. Feel free to add as many veggies as you like!

PREP TIME: **30 MINUTES**   YIELD: **1 SERVING**

¼ cup sweet potato
½ cup quinoa
1 cup water
1 handful leafy greens
½ avocado
Carrots, chopped
Cucumber, chopped
Hemp seeds
Squeeze of lemon juice
Drizzle of tahini

Chop and roast the sweet potato for 20 minutes at 400°.
Add the quinoa and water to a saucepan and bring to a boil.
Once boiling, reduce to low heat and cover with a lid for 15 minutes until done. Top your base of leafy greens with the precooked sweet potato and quinoa. Add avocado to your liking and then the chopped carrots and cucumber. Sprinkle with hemp seeds and drizzle lemon juice and tahini on top.

12

GROW YOUR *Patience*

GOOD THINGS TAKE TIME. You and I have heard this before and have probably been annoyed by it, but it is true. Think about this: Planting an apple seed and expecting to taste a delicious apple a week later is unrealistic. Eating salads and doing squats for three days and expecting to see results immediately is not realistic. If we view patience as a prize rather than something to be avoided, our perspectives and our experiences will shift for the better.

Proverbs 14:23 says, "In all labor there is profit." This means that your ten-minute workout counts. And not only does it count, but you will reap profit from it! Hold on to this verse the next time you're ready to throw in the towel after not seeing the fruit of your labor. It's growing. You will reap what you sow. We are so quick to become discouraged while we're growing.

The farmer doesn't get to tell the tree on what day it will produce fruit. The tree simply grows. The rain comes. The sun beats down. The seed even has to die before it grows. And then after many days, months, years, the tree not only produces one apple but becomes a giant apple tree capable of creating more delicious pieces of fruit. The seed did not complain when the storm rolled in. When the rain poured, the soil soaked it in. When the wind blew, the roots grew deep.

God is doing the same thing with us. He's growing us. He knows and sees a storm's ultimate good. He knows challenges will inspire patience, which will do its perfect work and bear fruit that is sweeter. My friend, there is profit in all labor. Do not give up—good things take time.

GOD WILL GROW YOU

Our motivation is stirred and regenerated in the hope of God's timing. Have you bumped up against doubt or a physical setback? A spiritual one? God is growing you. Psalm 1:3 says, "He shall be like a tree planted by the rivers of water, that brings forth its fruit in its season, whose leaf also shall not wither; and whatever he does shall prosper." The tree isn't just good for its fruit. Even in the off-seasons, it's providing blessings and benefits. It's a place for little kids to climb, explore, and imagine. It becomes a shelter of refreshing shade on a hot day. It's a work of art with brilliantly painted leaves, inspiring awe in every passerby.

Before the tree offers great fruit, the seed doesn't worry about how it's going to produce the fruit. And fruit doesn't force itself to grow; it simply abides. Working out should be something you want to do, not something you force yourself to do or worry about. Take the pressure off yourself to produce! Produce! Produce!

Take a breath. Abide in God and His time line for you, trusting that in due season, you will reap what you sow, and enjoy the profit of your labor. Let's not forget how beautiful the growing seasons are even before the harvest. When you're not seeing fruit, it is a time for your roots to grow deep and strong. Before God brings us into all the promises He has for us, He will refine us from the inside out—and patience is what He often uses.

So don't give up. Your workout counts. Your rest days count. Let go of your time line and trust in the One who created sunrises and sunsets. Savor the beauty of abiding instead of striving. Don't try to rush out ahead because you'll miss what God is

> Take a breath. Abide in God and His time line for you, trusting that in due season, you will reap what you sow, and enjoy the profit of your labor.

trying to do in you now. Don't grow tired or "become sluggish, but imitate those who through faith and patience inherit the promises" (Hebrews 6:12). You will grow as you rest in His time line for your life. Beautiful things take time. And you, my friend, are God's most beautiful thing.

ACTION STEP

This sounds crazy, but work out today without music. With every movement, tell yourself that you're strong and you can do it. Feel each contraction and focus on your mind-muscle connection.

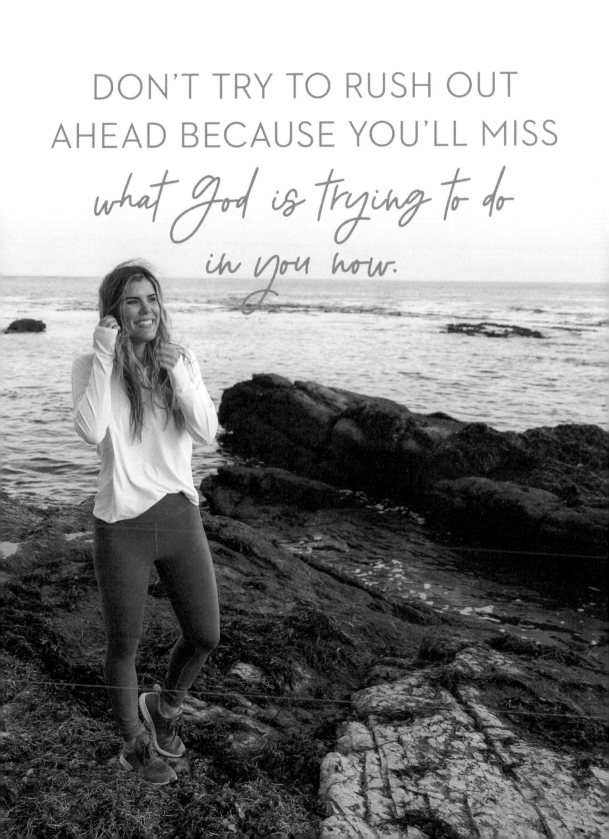

DON'T TRY TO RUSH OUT
AHEAD BECAUSE YOU'LL MISS
*what god is trying to do
in you now.*

13

SET REALISTIC
Goals

HONESTLY, AS GLAMOROUS AS LIVING an active lifestyle sounds, it comes with lots of sweat and not so much sparkle. Most days I don't really feel like working out. The secrets to motivation are straightforward: Set realistic goals, don't wait until you feel like doing something to do it, and put one foot in front of the other.

In his book *Finish,* author Jon Acuff observes that we tend to fail because we super-size our goals due to our pursuit of perfectionism. And most of us would get far more done if we cut our initial goal in half. [1]

I have found this to be true: Getting something—anything—done is motivating!

PLAN FOR SUCCESS

If you want to work out and live healthy, then try this strategy to set realistic goals:

1. Make a plan that fits into your day. Don't shape a workout routine or a food-prep plan that won't fit into your daily schedule. Get real about what will work.

2. Squish "perfect" like it's your full-time job. The enemy to productivity is perfection. When I meet with someone who is struggling, they are often stalled

---

1 Jon Acuff, *Finish* (New York: Portfolio / Penguin Books, 2018), 20.

Move. Make it fun. And get it done.

by perfectionism and don't realize it. Until it is pointed out, they don't notice that their short list of expectations is really a list of required perfections that will work against them.

3. Get rid of those "rules" that are illusions getting in your way. Truth. You don't have to work out in the morning. You don't have to burn a certain number of calories for it to "count" as a workout. You don't have to wear a certain kind of exercise outfit to go to the gym. You just do it! Move. Make it fun. And get it done.

4. Do something every day. My workouts this week have ranged from 10 minutes to more than 30 minutes, but every day, I did something. It doesn't matter if I did every workout perfectly or worked out for a set amount of time. I did it—I moved—and that's what matters.

5. Take one step. Full disclosure here: I love working out once I'm doing it. I get this rush in the middle of my workout when I'm dripping with sweat. Before the workout…that's a different story. To stay healthy, I follow my own advice and take one step. Then another. I pray and ask God to help me do what it takes for me to honor my body. Some days that's resting, but some days that's working out. On the workout days when I'm less motivated, I don't overthink it, I simply put on my leggings and lace up my shoes. Then I take a literal next step and head into the garage. Then I turn on the music. Then I do active stretches. And then I do the first move. Then the next.

Soon I'm into the workout. The dread goes away and the enjoyment rushes in! You are capable of this as well. Every day, ask God to help you honor the body He's given you, and then take the next step. I promise, it makes things a whole lot simpler.

ACTION STEP

Get ten minutes of sunlight on bare skin first thing in the morning to boost vitamin D and help reset your circadian rhythm.

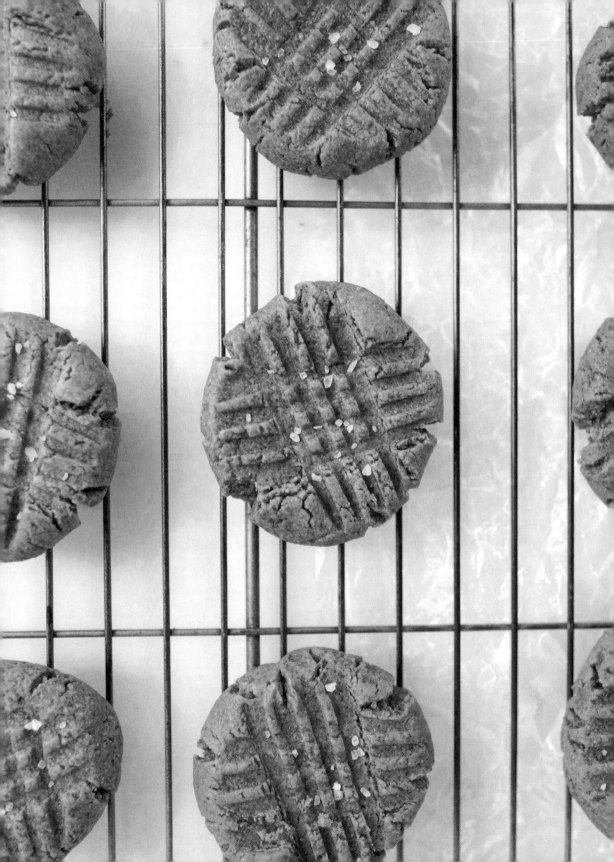

THE BEST PEANUT BUTTER COOKIES

These cookies might be the easiest and most delicious cookies you'll ever make. They are tasty, made with wholesome ingredients, and take under 15 minutes from start to finish. What could be better than that?

PREP TIME: 15 MINUTES   YIELD: 14 COOKIES

1 cup peanut butter
1 cup coconut sugar
1 egg

Mix all ingredients until combined. Scoop out spoonfuls of dough onto a parchment paper lined baking sheet and bake for 8 minutes at 350°.

Optional: Sprinkle with chunky salt!

14

CHANGE
Your Days

IF YOU WANT TO CHANGE YOUR LIFE, CHANGE YOUR DAYS. If we couple that motivation with what Jesus said, "Do not worry about tomorrow, for tomorrow will worry about its own things" (Matthew 6:34), then I think we have a formula for a beautiful life. Focus on today, do your best, and leave the rest up to God.

I recently read that a member of one of my favorite Christian bands writes a song every day. As in, *Every. Single. Day.* Why am I telling you this? Because what we do every day counts. Instead of worrying about how to change your whole life, start living well today. The English bishop Joseph Hall is credited with saying, "Every day is a little life, and our whole life is but a day repeated. Therefore, live every day as if it would be the last."

Do you want to get healthy? Do you want to eat well? Do you want to wake up early and spend time with God? Do you want to use your God-given gifts to the fullest potential? Of course, you do, and I'm right there with you. The good news is that God has given you today. And He told you not to worry about tomorrow.

How do others accomplish great things? Did your favorite author quit after writing one page? Did your doctor graduate school by taking one class? No. They started with

> ## Whatever you want to do, ask God to help you take the first step today.

that first step and kept on going. I personally have to commit right away or it won't happen. If I say I want to spend time in my Bible daily but put it off until I have more time tomorrow, I'll never make the time. Instead of worrying about how you're going to run a whole marathon, just run a mile today. God has given you the gift of today.

YOUR DAYS ADD UP

Our life is the sum of our days, so we ought to make our days count. One of my favorite verses to hold in my mind and heart is Proverbs 14:23 because it says that there is profit in all labor. Did you hear that? All labor! Yes, that means your ten-minute workout! You reap the reward of energy and the endorphin high that God created our bodies with. Yes, that even means when I bake chocolate chip cookies for Bo, there is a reward—the reward of a delicious cookie and a happy husband (and I'm happy too).

You won't make the evening news or start trending online because you spent time with God or did the dishes or took care of your body. But there are internal and eternal rewards for being faithful in the little things that only you and God see. It's a good day, my friend, when you hit the pillow and know in your heart, "I walked with my God today, I took care of the body He has given me. I was a good steward over my home. I took a step toward the dream He put on my heart, and I was faithful with my today." That's all we can do—live today well. And by the grace of God, we will.

ACTION STEP

Today try to eat a vegetable with every meal. Throw a handful of spinach into your smoothie. Snack on raw veggies and make them a side dish with tonight's dinner.

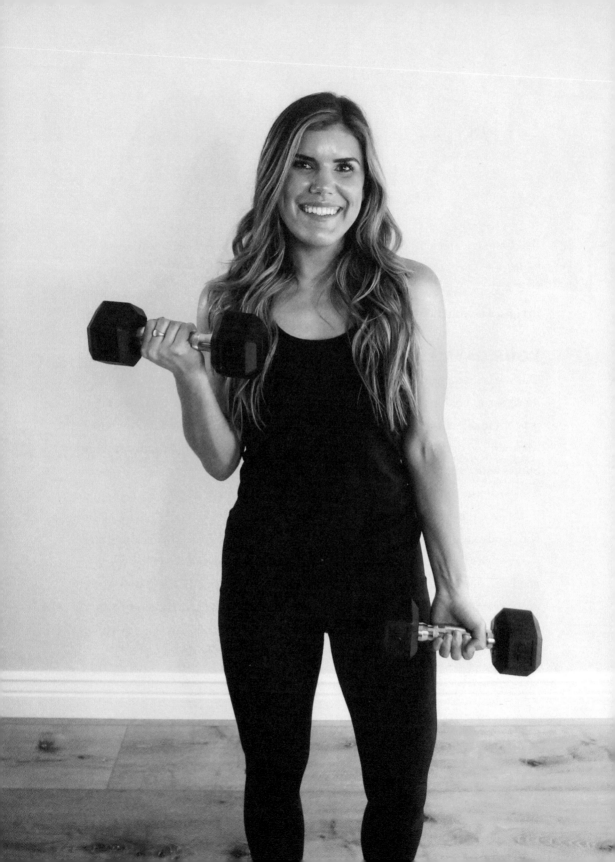

THREE WAYS TO HAVE MORE CONSISTENT WORKOUTS

Keep this in mind: If I like what I do, I'll follow through. Now make a plan.

1. MAKE IT FUN TO GET IT DONE.

Choose activities that motivate and challenge you but don't bore you. If going to a gym is unappealing, buy hand weights and work out to an online program. Play tennis. Go on a hike. Take an energetic dog for a walk or jog in the park.

2. MAKE IT A DATE.

When I set healthy strength goals leading up to my wedding, I trained with my future sister-in-law. Every week I looked forward to laughing and putting in some sweat equity with her. Ask a friend or find a workout pal by posting online, in your church bulletin, or at the gym.

3. RETHINK YOUR "WHY."

Our bodies are to be appreciated. I used to work out hard to "correct" the shape of my legs. One day someone I knew became paralyzed from the waist down. As I prayed for them, I was convicted for my distorted view of the human body. We're whole beings in Christ no matter what our physical dwelling looks like. My workouts became motivated by thanksgiving, not perfection. If you've had physical trauma, experienced setbacks, or judged or rejected a part of you, ask for a healed perspective. Move forward in your healthy why.

When you shift your mindset from "have to" to "want to," you'll discover the joy of a healthy lifestyle that nurtures your body, soul, and mind.

15

KEEP
Stepping

YOU ONLY HAVE TODAY, SO WHAT ARE YOU GOING TO DO WITH IT?
Are you going to put off the dreams God places on your heart until everything is perfect or are you going to take a step toward them? Believe me, I understand how easy it is to delay starting a task, a plan, or even a desire of the heart.

It took me three years to get my certification in personal training. Did it really take me three years? Nope. It took only three months of studying and preparation. So why did I drag it out for so long? Because I was waiting for the perfect time. I wanted to get certified so badly but it never seemed like the right time to start studying. When I did start to study, I felt overwhelmed and behind. Then one day, I woke up and decided that if I didn't take at least one step to reach my goal that day, I was never going to. It's about finishing every day satisfied that you took a step toward your goal. Not a million steps. Just one step.

Earlier I wrote out four simple steps to take on the days when you don't want to work out. The idea of making slow but sure progress works for most any area of life, including something as important as getting an education or finishing a long-desired goal.

Take a step forward today. Don't wait
for an ideal day in the near future to
start your healthy lifestyle.

What that meant for my situation was studying all day long sometimes. On other days I went over practice tests while waiting in the car before church because that was the best step I could take that day. I made progress through slow and steady measures. It doesn't matter that I did things differently than other people or even than what I had originally planned. I did it. And I finished strong.

YOUR VERSION OF FINISHING STRONG

Some days finishing strong will be crawling into bed knowing you crushed your workout and anticipating how sore you'll be the next morning. Some days it will be freely eating a cupcake without guilt because you stopped believing the lies. Other days finishing strong will be walking your dog around the block because that's all the energy you have for that day. Some days you'll finish strong by resting.

Take a step forward today. Don't wait for an ideal day in the near future to start your healthy lifestyle. And definitely don't wait until you feel like it. Just take one step.

You finish strong only if you've actually started the journey! And today requires nothing more than your participation. Keep it simple. Wake up every single day and determine to take single steps in the right direction. I'm writing this to remind you that God has a good future planned for you. I know this because that's what He promises in His Word. I also know that your life might feel too heavy for you, simply too heavy for you to carry on your own. Begin "casting all your care upon Him, for He cares for you" (1 Peter 5:7). Ask God to give you inner rest down deep in your soul, and remember, "You do not have because you do not ask" (James 4:2).

The enemy wants you bound by discouragement and defeat. But you are fighting from victory, not for victory, because Jesus has already won. Ask God to give you the endurance you need to run in this race of life. When you feel weary, wait on the Lord; He promises to renew your strength (Isaiah 40:31). Don't worry about your future; remember who holds the future. Just watch and see the blessings that God has in store for you as you remain on track with Him!

ACTION STEP

Slowly sip your coffee or tea this morning. With every sip you take, whisper a prayer of something you're thankful for to the Giver of good gifts.

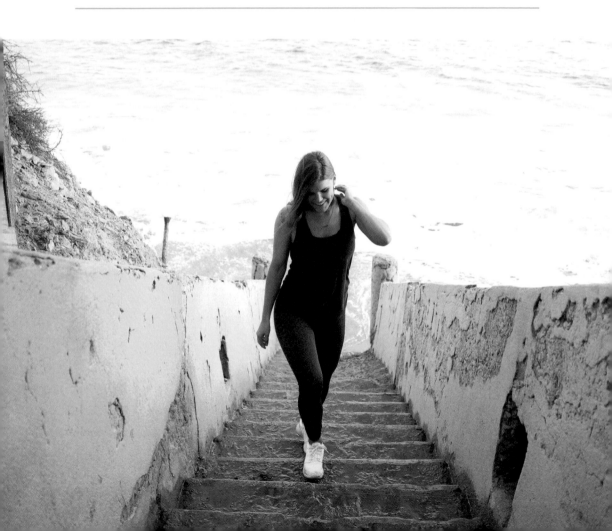

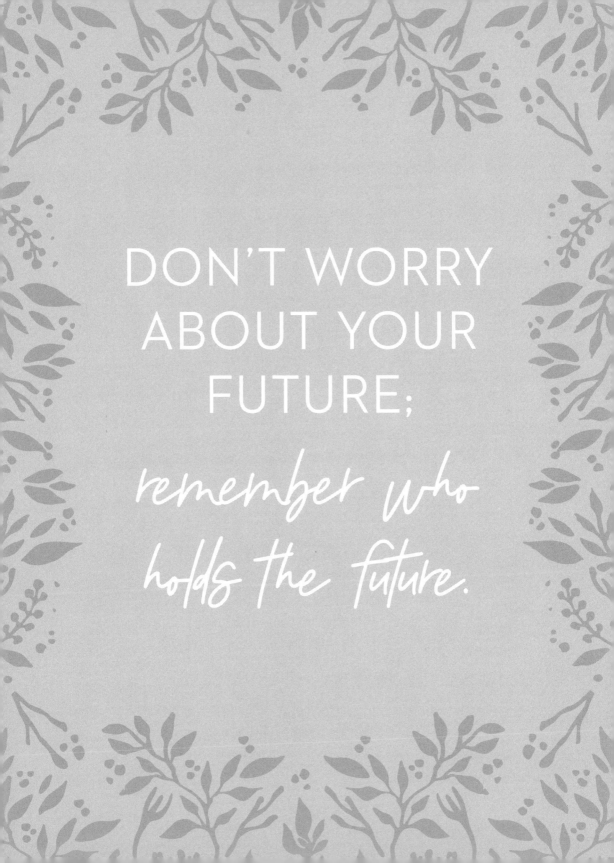

DON'T WORRY
ABOUT YOUR
FUTURE;

remember who
holds the future.

DON'T
PROVE IT—
Live It

HAVE YOU EVER FELT THE NEED to prove yourself to others or even to God? What area do you most often use to justify or establish your value?

finances

career

physical fitness

relationships

beauty

academics

popularity

_____ (What else do you turn to for validation?)

What does this have to do with motivation? A lot. Your response is likely acting as your main motivation for striving and earning value. There are tempting forces all around us, convincing us to seek identity through actions. I've faced these and given in to them countless times.

In Christ, we can resist the temptations to prove our eternal value through world-approved achievements and standards.

What you might not know is that Jesus faced the same temptation as well.

When Satan was tempting Jesus, he said to Him, "If You are the Son of God, command that these stones become bread" (Matthew 4:3). The Greek word for "if" that is being used here means "indeed." Satan was saying, "Indeed You are the Son of God, so command that these stones become bread." You see, Satan wasn't doubting Jesus's identity; he just wanted Jesus to prove His identity. He was basically saying, "You need to do something of real worth to prove who You are."

Jesus could have demonstrated His power to squelch Satan's taunt. But He didn't need to. The temptation didn't spark motivation in Jesus to prove who He was because His identity was and is secure. It's the same for us. When our identity is in Christ, we can resist the temptations to prove our eternal value through world-approved achievements and standards. The times I've given in were the times I wasn't resting in my identity as God's beloved daughter.

BECOME NEW

The enemy desires to see you striving to prove that you are the daughter of God, but don't fall into that trap! We are accepted only because of Jesus. All we need to do is to accept the work that His Son did on the cross. You can't earn what is already yours, and there's no need to prove what is true!

The next time you feel pressured to justify your worth, stop and recall this verse:

Therefore, if anyone is in Christ, he is a new creation; old things have passed away; behold, all things have become new. 2 CORINTHIANS 5:17

Spend your days motivated, secure, and strong as a new creation in Christ and as a treasured daughter who confidently stands on and acts from her identity. This is how you glorify God. When you stop running in circles to prove your worth, you can start improving your life physically and spiritually.

The next time you walk into a workout or sit down to plan your weekly meals, approach the adventure as a new creation.

ACTION STEP

When you're tempted to spend money on a new workout outfit, put those earnings toward trying a new class, like barre or group fitness training.

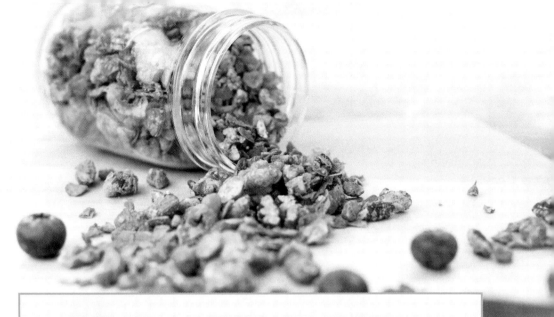

GRAIN-FREE GRANOLA

My husband, Bo, and I think this crunchy, healthy granola is much better than store-bought.

PREP TIME: **30 MINUTE**   YIELD: **6 SERVINGS**

½ cup walnuts
½ cup almonds
¼ cup pecans
¼ cup cashews
1 cup coconut flakes
(unsweetened)

½ tsp. cinnamon
½ cup blanched almond flour
¼ cup maple syrup
Pinch of salt

Chop the nuts to the desired bite size. Mix the dry ingredients until well combined. Pour the maple syrup over the dry ingredients and mix well. Pour the granola onto a baking sheet covered with parchment paper. Bake at 325° for 15 minutes. Flip and stir the granola. Bake 5 more minutes. Remove from the oven and cool until room temperature. Enjoy with your Homemade Almond Milk (page 25).

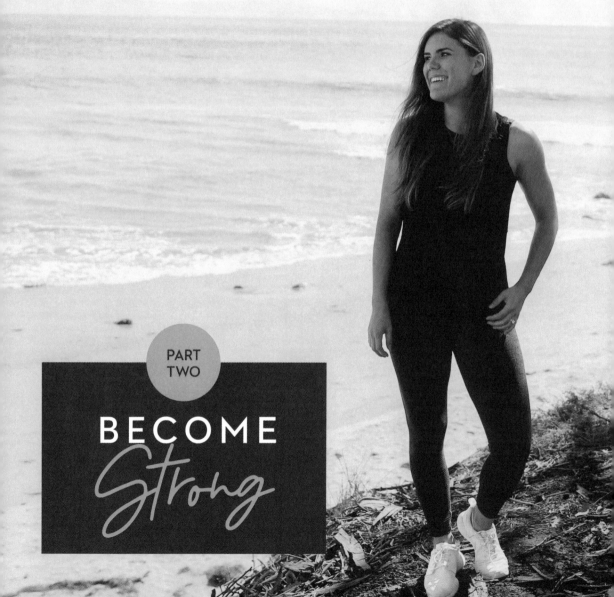

PART
TWO

BECOME
Strong

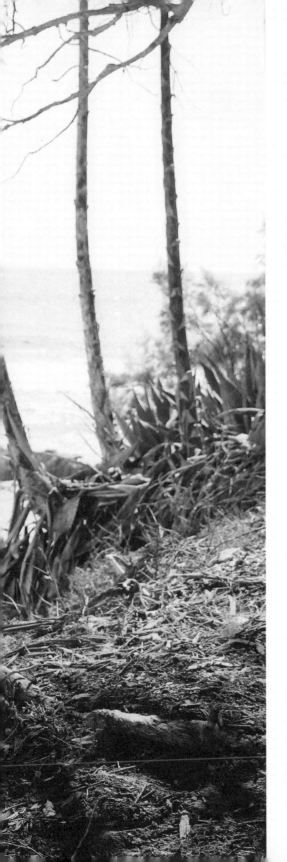

My gym membership card is scanned. I smile at the other early birds who aim for a saner, stronger day by caring for their bodies. I enter the weight-training room, and my spirit lightens at the sight of Jan, my longtime trainer. Her joyful personality and physically challenging workouts inspire me to be strong. But her encouragement reaches beyond my physical journey.

I had experienced God's acceptance through Jan's encouragement. Felt Jesus's unconditional love in her faithful greeting, "So glad you're here, Cambria."

During my years of binge eating, I hit an emotional low point. In my mom's bedroom, I hid from my family to devour ciabatta bread and honey with desperation after days of severe restricting. As I consumed piece after piece, my peace was swept away in the flood of insults that filled my mind as quickly as I filled my stomach. "I am disgusting. I'm so weak...so worthless!" I cried a prayer of tears, and God gave me the grace to move past that night and into a new, mercy-filled tomorrow.

Today, she waves back to me. I start to load the weights for the first exercise. I'm eager to push my muscles to new limits and feel empowered, balanced, and strong. Jan never has anything but encouragement to say. Her example shows me God's strength when I am at my weakest.

"So glad you're here, Cambria!" She beams.

"Me too," I say as happy tears form. "Me too."

No matter what goes on in our lives, you and I can lean into God's strength as we take steps to personally grow physically and spiritually strong.

17

GOD BUILDS YOUR INNER *Strength*

GOD, I'M SO SORRY FOR *idolizing my appearance and my body. Forgive me for seeking my value in something other than You and Your love for me. Thank You for Your grace.* This was my prayer during that rock-bottom day I mentioned in this section's opening.

While revisiting that moment is uncomfortable, I am aware that it was a catalyst for me to know God and His healing strength intimately. It's the day I "got it"—understood that my inner strength comes not from me but from God.

We are hard-pressed on every side, yet not crushed; we are perplexed, but not in despair; persecuted, but not forsaken; struck down, but not destroyed—always carrying about in the body the dying of the Lord Jesus, that the life of Jesus also may be manifested in our body . 2 CORINTHIANS 4:8-10

He rebuilds us with
His incorruptible strength.

That's some serious strength! It's also an assurance: We do not need to hide our weaknesses in shame but can see them as a way to lean on God and to give Him glory. We are strongest when we recognize that we can do nothing without God:

> *Therefore I will boast all the more gladly of my weaknesses, so that the power of Christ may rest upon me.* 2 CORINTHIANS 12:9 ESV

On that painful day, God met me in my weakness. His love replaced the heavy yoke of shame with the light cloak of grace. After my prayer, a sense of forgiveness washed over me like an early morning sunrise streaking through the window. It felt new. *I* felt new. I had hope.

TORN DOWN TO BE REBUILT

The fresh start didn't happen on a Monday or a January 1. It didn't happen when I decided to pick myself up by my bootstraps and start anew. It happened as I sat defeated on my mom's bed with tears streaming and a spiritual ache matching the physical one I had caused by eating. In our weakness, God is strong. I was fully awake to His power and assurance. I trusted that I was not being torn down and left alone.

When we are torn down by circumstances or even choices, God does not use our frailty against us. It is then that He is strong in us, and not only that, but in the pain of a breakdown, He rebuilds us with His incorruptible strength.

I turn to my training to better understand this through the lens of a physical strength workout. As your muscles get sore, or break down, during a workout, they are preparing to rebuild even stronger. With faith we step into the gym, ready to brave the pain, knowing we'll be sore today and strong tomorrow. In the same way, we can enter our weakness, our teardown moments and seasons of bearing the weight of pain, knowing that God's strength in us will increase...if we surrender.

The definition of strength according to the National Academy of Sports Medicine is "the ability of the neuromuscular system to produce internal tension to overcome an external load."[2] I read that definition while studying to get my personal training certification, and it struck a heart chord. It still inspires me in this moment, both for me and for you.

You have a strength inside of you that is able to overcome any external load that tries to lay itself upon your shoulders. You have the ability to stand firm during the fiercest storm. The force to push back against the lies that weigh you down. The grit to press on when you're being pressed down. Where does strength like this come from? Listen to the words of Jesus:

> *"My grace is sufficient for you, for My strength is made perfect in weakness."*
> 2 CORINTHIANS 12:9

ACTION STEP
Make time today to play. Do something that makes your soul come alive.

---

2 National Academy of Sports Medicine, *NASM Essentials of Sports Performance Training*, rev. ed. (Burlington, MA: Jones & Bartlett Learning, 2014), 312.

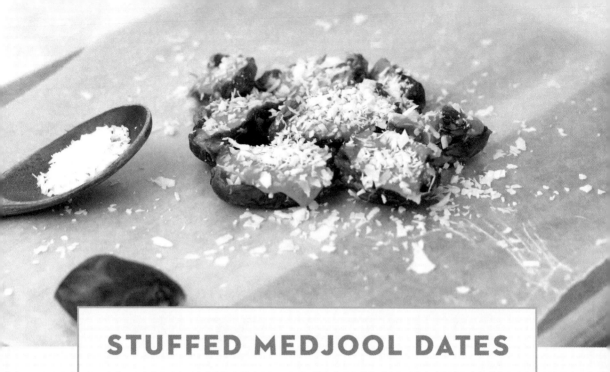

STUFFED MEDJOOL DATES

Packed with nutrients, dates are a perfect pre- or postworkout snack and taste like candy from above! It's a good thing they can be made in two minutes...you and friends will want more.

PREP TIME: **5 MINUTES**   YIELD: **1 SERVING**

---

2 or 3 Medjool dates (remove seeds)
2 or 3 T. almond butter
2 or 3 T. coconut flakes

Stuff each date with 1 tablespoon of almond butter.
Sprinkle with coconut flakes.

18

CORE WORKOUTS FOR BODY *and Soul*

TODAY WE'RE GOING TO FOCUS on your core strength—physical and spiritual.

Let me explain this in a practical, personal trainer kind of way. You need to start off by strengthening your inner core before you move on to bigger and better workouts. We'll start with the physical core.

Your inner core muscles attach directly to your spine. As you strengthen your glutes, low back, and abs, you create a stable center that secures you for larger strength moves, activities, or everyday demands such as sitting in front of your laptop for hours. I didn't know this when I first started working out. I went for the big exercises, the obvious sweat-inducers. Neglecting your foundation can lead to all kinds of muscle imbalances.

Most people don't want to do core work because it is boring. It doesn't require heavier weights or intense, upbeat workout music to keep you "in the zone." And it certainly isn't visually impressive. Nope. Some of the best core workouts are subtle and involve lying on your back while doing slow glute pulses awkwardly in the gym as everyone walks by. Recent scene at my fitness center: a guy next to me repeatedly trying to initiate a conversation while I'm doing booty bridges on the floor, wearing headphones, and minding my own business. I have nothing to say but *awkward*.

If you start out your physical fitness program with gusto to work only the large, obvious muscles without developing the inner muscles, you'll end up injured, off-balance, and discouraged. You need to build a firm foundation. Core before more.

DEVELOP THAT SPIRITUAL CORE

When was the last time you did something that makes your soul happy? Physical fitness and eating well are great, but sometimes the most important things can be overlooked. When it comes to developing a spiritual core, we also need subtle reinforcements and strength building.

The Bible says, "Pleasant words are like a honeycomb, sweetness to the soul and health to the bones" (Proverbs 16:24). If that's true, and it is, then you can bet the exact opposite is true: Bitter words can sour your soul and rot your bones. Remember Proverbs 14:30? It says that envy does that very thing. And how does envy usually manifest? Personally, I generate a lot of negative thoughts about myself. The greener I am with envy, the more black-and-white my views become: *That girl is so perfect. I am the total opposite. I am a mess.*

Emotions and circumstances can sway our states of mind, injure our spirits and attitudes, and throw us off balance. That is, unless we have a strong core of truth. A strong foundation of belief in our worth is essential for our stability.

We create this foundation by developing our identity in Christ. The influence of our positive self-talk doesn't come close to the power of our identity-in-Christ talk. I know that you know that. Vulnerable honest moment here: Think about the time you tried to put on your jeans and nearly cried because they didn't get past your thighs. The negative thoughts start because you are discouraged—that pair of jeans fit two months ago but is now destined for your unwearable drawer.

Is the Instagram post that says, "You're beautiful! Believe it!" going to change the way you feel right now? Probably not. It's true—you *are* beautiful, and you should believe it. But by this point, you've thrown those jeans across the floor and vowed to never wear real pants again. #sweatpantsforlife. I know because I've been there.

It takes great strength to speak to your soul and heart with God's love and grace. Not only can our words be sweet and pleasant, but the book of Proverbs says that our words have the power of life and death (Proverbs 18:21).

We develop those abilities through subtle exercises: "Let the words of my mouth and the meditation of my heart be acceptable in Your sight, O Lord, my strength and my Redeemer" (Psalm 19:14). Meditating on God's Word won't initially look and feel like it is doing as much as the more "grand" spiritual exercises like preaching or participating in a Bible study; it will be a quiet, subtle workout that changes you from deep within. Start your spiritual core workout today by reading these truths slowly and deliberately:

- We are fearfully and wonderfully made (Psalm 139:14).
- God has a good plan for our lives (Philippians 1:6).
- We are loved and heard (Psalm 86:5).
- We are forgiven when we confess our sins (1 John 1:9).

My advice? To build the inner strength that comes from the Lord and your identity in Him, do three sets of ten reps of this spiritual core workout daily.

ACTION STEP

Take ten minutes to clean out and organize your fitness wardrobe today. Donate clothes that no longer fit and organize your tops, leggings, and shorts so you can easily find the right workout outfit for your exercise today.

THE INFLUENCE OF OUR

positive self-talk

DOESN'T COME CLOSE

TO THE POWER OF OUR

identity-in-Christ talk.

19

TRUST

Resistance Training

READY FOR A STRENGTH-TRAINING LESSON? Okay. Class is in session. Don't worry...no exams and no getting up to speak in front of the entire class. This is a cool lesson that blends our interests in the physical and spiritual ways to become strong. God strong.

First, do you remember that strength is the ability to internally overcome an external load? Okay, that was the only quiz, and I gave you the answer. Painless.

TWO PARTS TO STRENGTH

Today, we are going to look at the way a muscle responds to that external load and how there are two parts to muscle movement, both of which build strength:

- The concentric action of the muscle is when the muscle is being shortened. For example, do a bicep curl right now. The muscle is contracted and tight.
- The eccentric action is when the muscle is being lengthened. This is when you release the bicep curl and slowly straighten your arm.

When we're being obedient in difficult times,
God is stretching and strengthening us.
We feel weak but we're becoming strong.

Most people think of the concentric action as the difficult part of the muscle movement and, therefore, the part that builds strength. But what they don't realize is that we're getting stronger even in the eccentric movement. That lengthening, stretching, and waiting that feels so long before you do another rep is doing something quite productive.

My strength coach used to say, "Work the negative!" The negative is the eccentric part of the muscle contraction. It's not going against the resistance to become stronger—it's going with the resistance. In our faith journey, we are going along with the resistance when we say yes to seasons of waiting and difficulty. When we're being obedient in difficult times, God is stretching and strengthening us. We feel weak but we're becoming strong.

Now, on the flip side, the concentric is going against the resistance—the weight—so we feel the pressure more significantly. In our acceptance and growth journey, this kind of growth manifests when we look in the mirror and push against the need to "fix" or criticize something we see. We press on through the weight of perfection, the judgment of others, our negative self-talk, or the heft of society's standards, and we hold steady in God's strength. We're empowered in truth.

The takeaway is this: Be still and wait for the Lord to strengthen you. Be steadfast as He stretches you and strengthens you. And when you are bearing the weight and moving against resistance, trust that His truth will sustain you and hold you up.

Class dismissed! My favorite class was PE anyway.

ACTION STEP

Tonight when you go to bed, practice intentionl breathing. It will help you wind down for a good night's rest.

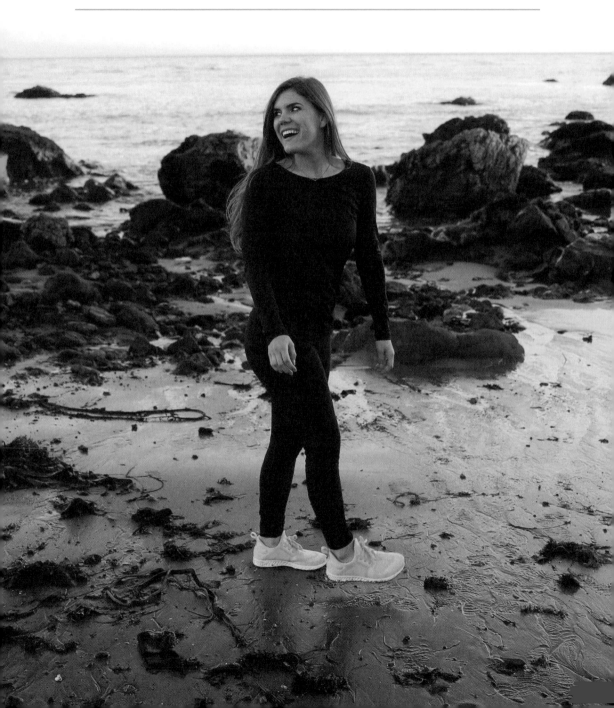

BELIEVE YOU'RE STRONG AND WONDERFULLY MADE

Nourish your soul with promises God has spoken over you!
Find a cozy chair or a bench with a view, and savor these
truths about your strength and wonder in the Lord.

You are altogether beautiful,
my darling; there is no flaw in you.

SONG OF SOLOMON 4:7 NIV

I praise you, for I am fearfully
and wonderfully made.

PSALM 139:14 ESV

She is clothed with strength and dignity;
she can laugh at the days to come.

PROVERBS 31:25 NIV

We are God's masterpiece.

EPHESIANS 2:10 NLT

You made all the delicate, inner
parts of my body and knit me
together in my mother's womb.

PSALM 139:13 NLT

Behold, God is my salvation; I will trust,
and will not be afraid; for the LORD
GOD is my strength and my song, and
he has become my salvation.

ISAIAH 12:2 ESV

I'm so thankful that I don't have to rely on my own strength.
I'll come to You for rest and refreshment every day as I ask
for You to hold and protect my heart. I will lean into Your
strength as I am becoming strong physically, spiritually,
and mentally. In Jesus's name, amen.

20

CHANGE YOUR MIND, CHANGE YOUR *Direction*

IMAGINE YOU AND I ARE WORKOUT PARTNERS, and someone who has never worked out before instructs us to do a specific, intense arm routine for three weeks. Over that time period, a pain in our shoulders develops and becomes worse with each session. But we stubbornly keep at it. By week five, we're both too injured to do anything. We caused damage by sticking with the initial choice and by paying attention to someone who didn't have our best interest at heart.

That seems a little crazy. Would we really do that? Now think of a life circumstance in which you struggle and encounter frustration or even emotional pain. What started you on that path? Was there an initial point when you started to listen to advice that wasn't given with your interest and health as a priority? Maybe it started because you listened to your own lies and kept telling yourself the situation would change even if you did not.

This happens, right? It does in my life. It is surprisingly easy to get sidetracked or derailed from truth. Circumstances, fear, change, and even success can turn our focus from God's truth. We end up going the wrong direction.

In comes repentance.

The word "repentance" sounds so harsh to most of us today. It isn't exactly a topic we throw around in casual conversation, is it? But maybe it should be. I want to look at it in a new light so we understand its power for our pursuit of body and soul health.

Jesus calls us to repent, which simply means to change our mind, change direction so we can follow Him. To do a 180 in your mind, to turn from one way of thinking and go the other way. Toward Him. Toward the eternal hope of His love. Toward our purpose and wholeness. Repentance is essential in those times when we're following unhealthy behaviors, thoughts, or beliefs.

If we're going the way of self-pity, self-indulgence, or self-destruction, we need to shift to face a completely different direction: "And do not be conformed to this world, but be transformed by the renewing of your mind, that you may prove what is that good and acceptable and perfect will of God" (Romans 12:2). Our lives are shaped by our thoughts. That's why we're told to fix our minds on things above, walk by faith not by sight, repent, and renew our minds.

Jesus says, "Brood of vipers! How can you, being evil, speak good things? For out of the abundance of the heart the mouth speaks" (Matthew 12:34). If the words that come from our mouths flow from our hearts, we should do what Jesus says and keep our hearts with all diligence. We do this by following the guidance of Paul: "Finally, brethren, whatever things are true, whatever things are noble, whatever things are just, whatever things are pure, whatever things are lovely, whatever things are of good report, if there is any virtue and if there is anything praiseworthy—meditate on these things" (Philippians 4:8).

Notice that Paul starts off his list with things that are true. When we focus on what is true, we're able to recognize the lies much faster and avoid being ensnared by them.

Are we going TO GO our way OR god's way?

REPENT. REPEAT.

Every time an intrusive thought enters your mind, quote or read Scripture to fix your mind on truth. Hebrews 4:12 says, "For the word of God is living and powerful, and sharper than any two-edged sword, piercing even to the division of soul and spirit, and of joints and marrow, and is a discerner of the thoughts and intents of the heart." Do you recall when we explored how God fights for us? Well, His Word fights for us too. It's able to combat the lies that try to lead us away from the truth of God.

When we repent and bring falsehoods to God's presence in prayer, God's truth renews our minds and gives us the strength and power to fight the next deception or discouragement. We don't have to fall victim to mind games when we have the power of God's Word on our side. We don't need to live a fearful, depressed, anxious, worried life full of self-pity when we can ask God to help us set our minds on Him. When we do so, we live lives of victory, as those who overcome. Repentance is powerful because it ultimately determines our eternal destiny. Are we going to go our way or God's way?

Romans 8:6 reminds us where real life is found: "To be carnally minded is death, but to be spiritually minded is life and peace." Remember the old hymn, "Turn your eyes upon Jesus, look full in His wonderful face, And the things of earth will grow strangely dim, In the light of His glory and grace." When we turn to look to Jesus and His truths, we change direction, and we move forward in faith and peace toward the true story God is telling through our lives.

Ask God to help you meditate on things that are true, noble, just, pure, lovely, of good report, virtuous, and praiseworthy, and experience how your life transforms.

ACTION STEP ────────────────────────

Go outside today. Even if it's only for five minutes, sunshine and fresh air are good for the soul.

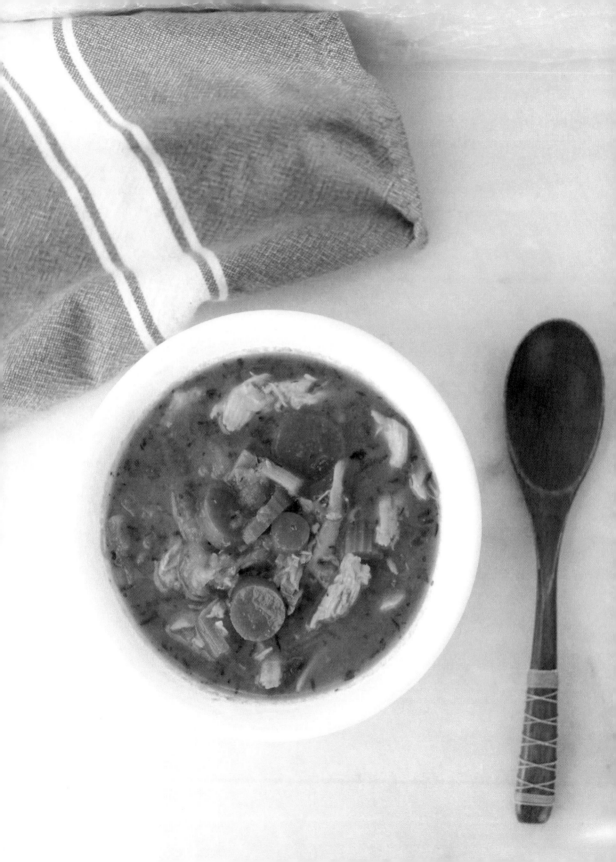

IMMUNITY-BOOST CHICKEN SOUP

This is my favorite soup to make. It's bursting with flavor, and the garlic and turmeric are great immunity boosters to keep you healthy year-round.

PREP TIME: 1.5 HOURS   YIELD: 8 SERVINGS

1½ cups chicken breast or tenderloins, cooked and shredded

3 carrots

2 stalks celery

1 sweet onion

1 T. avocado oil

2 tsp. arrowroot flour

2 tsp. dried turmeric

1 tsp. dried thyme

1 tsp. dried basil

¼ tsp. dried oregano

½ tsp. paprika

½ tsp. onion powder

½ tsp. garlic powder

2 garlic cloves, fresh-pressed

Salt to taste

Pepper to taste

1 (32 oz.) carton chicken broth

1 cup water

1 T. ghee

Preheat your oven to 350° and bake the chicken for 18 to 20 minutes. Let the chicken cool and shred it with a fork or an electric mixer. Chop the carrot, celery, and onion into small bits. Sauté them in the avocado oil over medium heat in a large pot. Add the arrowroot powder to thicken. Add the spices and continue to cook over medium heat. Mix in the chicken broth and water, and bring to a boil for 15 minutes. Add the ghee and the chicken. Turn down to low heat, cover, and let simmer for 40 minutes. Enjoy!

21

FEED YOUR
Hunger

IF WE WANT STRONG BODIES, we need to continually serve them with nutritious food. If we want to grow strong in the Lord, we need to continually feed our spirits with His Word. Jesus said in Matthew 4:4, "It is written, 'Man shall not live by bread alone, but by every word that proceeds from the mouth of God.'" So let me ask you this: Do you really believe what Jesus is saying about another kind of food?

Picture this: You're driving in your car while drinking a smoothie when you realize you're all out of gas. Instead of making your way to the gas station you pull over, hop out, and begin to pour your smoothie into your gas tank. This is dumb. And this is definitely not going to work. Why? Because you just poured puréed strawberries instead of gasoline into your vehicle.

Cars need gas. Bodies need food. Souls need truth.

The bread of the world is not going to fuel our soul strength. We need specific "fuels" for the specific aspects of our being. Learning to know what to put into our souls and our bodies takes time and a willingness to learn.

The Word of God provides the only nourishment for your soul on this planet.

WHEN THE HUNGER COMES

When I am very hungry, I become agitated, angry. Hangry, you know? Typically, I don't allow myself to get to such a miserable state. I eat. I snack. And when I feel the hunger coming on, I stop whatever I'm doing, and my attention goes into getting food. How often do we stop whatever we're doing to pray? Or wake up every single morning eager to feed on God's Word? Have you ever thought about nourishment in this way?

When you're aiming for fitness goals, you'll be tempted to focus only on eating the right food and exercising. But nourishing your body and neglecting your spirit is going to leave you hungry and malnourished in all areas of your life. You can't live on protein bars alone!

We know this from experience: We can't give our all during a workout if we haven't eaten all day. We can't give our all in our lives, relationships, partnerships with God, and spiritual training if we haven't feasted on spiritually satisfying food.

Are you spiritually hungry? You need the bread of life: God's Word. You need time with Jesus. You know how you grab a banana or blend up a smoothie to take on the go when your mornings are rushed? Well, the same thing applies to your spiritual nourishment. Instead of rushing off in the morning—whether it's to go to work or to work out—carve out space for sacred feasting. Open the Bible and dig in. Jesus told the people to eat His body and drink His blood. The Bible says it was a hard saying for the people and that many turned to walk away from Jesus, since they thought He was talking about cannibalism. Jesus then turned to look at His disciples after many had left Him and asked them, "Do you also want to go away?" Peter then piped up and spoke some of the sweetest words in the whole Bible:

"Lord, to whom shall we go? You have the words of eternal life." JOHN 6:68

Jesus alone has those words. That's who we go to: the Bread of Life.

It is a beautiful, amazing fact that God is as close as your very breath. No matter where you are, you can be fed and satisfied. Talk to Him, walk with Him, and watch how you grow in Him as you taste and see that He is good through the living and active Word of God that provides the only nourishment for your soul on this planet.

ACTION STEP

Don't procrastinate today. Start the day off on the right foot by reading God's Word, journaling your prayers, and smashing a quick workout before you take on the rest of the day.

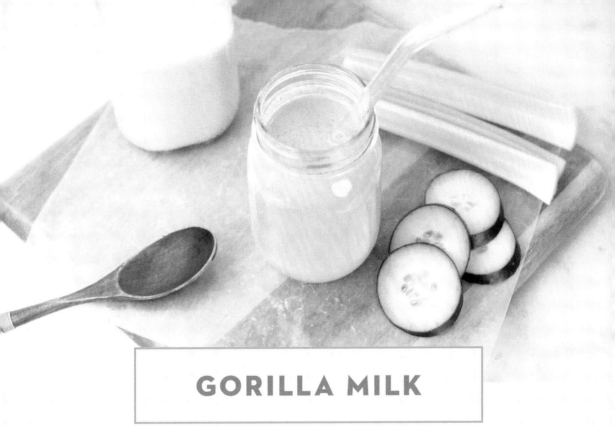

GORILLA MILK

Gorilla Milk is the perfect starter green juice if you're wanting to get into juicing but don't like the taste of greens. It's extremely hydrating and gives my skin a noticeable glow. It's mild in flavor and rich in nutrients.

PREP TIME: **5 MINUTE**   YIELD: **1 SERVING**

1 cucumber
1 cup spinach
1 stalk celery
1 cup Homemade Almond Milk (page 25)

Juice the vegetables and mix the fresh-pressed juice with the almond milk. Gorilla Milk is a recipe for glowing and radiant skin.

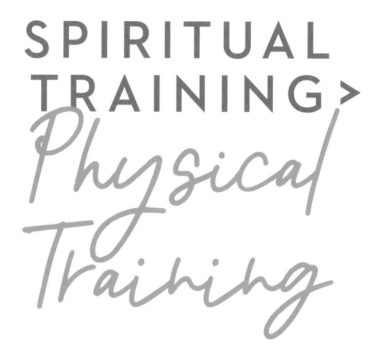

22

SPIRITUAL TRAINING >
Physical Training

BODILY EXERCISE PROFITS A LITTLE, but godliness is profitable for all things, having promise of the life that now is and of that which is to come" (1 Timothy 4:8). I love that this is in the Bible because it aligns my heart with what God thinks about temporal importance and eternal importance. (There are so many little details about life tucked within the pages of Scripture.) This verse directly says that bodily exercise gives us a profit; however, God is far more concerned with our spiritual strength than our physical strength.

Taking care of your body, which is the temple of the Holy Spirit, is honoring to God. But failing to take care of your spirit is neglecting to tend to what God considers to be of greater importance. I believe this verse is here to balance our loves. We

> Working out is a beautiful thing when our first love is Jesus because it allows us to serve our Lord rather than serve ourselves.

should love disciplining ourselves to be obedient to Christ more than disciplining our bodies in the gym.

I can tell you from personal experience that when I put my love for fitness above my love for Jesus, life gets pretty messy. Working out is a beautiful thing when our first love is Jesus because it allows us to serve our Lord rather than serve ourselves. When our bodies become our idols, we become earthly minded instead of heavenly minded. God calls us to have no other idols before Him. Our greatest devotion and affection should be for Jesus.

We can take inventory of our lives to see if we're motivated to be healthy for the glory of God rather than for our own glory. If fitness makes no room for faith, then we haven't found balance. Which actions are habits in your life? Your routines reveal where you invest your time and energy...and which area of life you are actively building as a discipline.

If you review the past month, were you more regularly seeking physical growth or spiritual growth? There's your answer.

WHERE DO YOU INVEST ENERGY?

Do you find that spending time with God in the morning conflicts with your workouts? I used to consistently make time for my favorite weight-training class, but I would skip doing what was most important for my soul: spending time with God. How much more important is it to care for your soul, which you will carry with you into eternity?

Exercise helps us take care of our bodies so we are able to serve the Lord with energy, but it needs to stay in the right place in our lives. Proverbs 31:17 says, "She girds herself with strength, and strengthens her arms." What does Proverbs 31 also say? "Charm is deceitful and beauty is passing, but a woman who fears the LORD, she shall be praised" (Proverbs 31:30). Simply put: We can strengthen our bodies, but real strength is found in a woman who fears the Lord.

Ask God to help you understand what 1 Timothy 4:8 looks like in your own life. What does it look like to strengthen your body and your spirit on the same day? Ask Him to guide you as you make a habit of doing your workouts and spending time with Him.

ACTION STEP

Next time you hit an afternoon slump, reach for an iced green tea and a handful of walnuts to give your brain a boost.

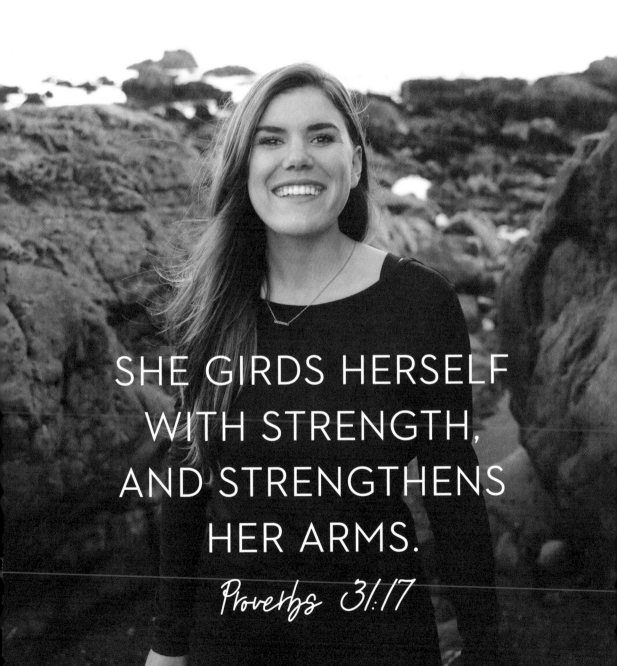

SHE GIRDS HERSELF
WITH STRENGTH,
AND STRENGTHENS
HER ARMS.

Proverbs 31:17

23

SEEK STRENGTH IN *Quietness*

AS I OPENED MY LAPTOP TO WRITE, I heard my husband's voice speak the words of Isaiah 30:7 (KJV) from the other room: "Their strength is to sit still." Bo is studying the Bible and likes to say verses aloud. That one sentence captured my heart. I kept listening. A few verses later, more words of great comfort wafted between rooms: "In returning and rest you shall be saved; in quietness and confidence shall be your strength" (Isaiah 30:15). Wow. Quietness. Strength in sitting still.

The world tells of a very different version of strength: strength as arriving at the top and being the best. I think it takes great strength to not be fixated on self-importance and power in a world that loves to sell perfection. I love what Mark Twain said about courage: "It is curious that physical courage should be so common in the world and moral courage so rare."

Where do we find moral courage and strength? By returning to quietness. By practicing stillness before the Lord. The world shames stillness as unprofitable. Oh, my. So much fruit is grown in the hidden gardens of our hearts when we take the time

Because our strength is found in sitting still in a restless world.

to sit quietly before Jesus in prayer. God loves you so much, and He is waiting for you to strengthen your heart in truth. In quietness. In His presence.

Your strength is everlasting when you tap into the greatest source of strength—Jesus Christ. Stillness will serve your commitment to mental, physical, emotional, and spiritual health and strength. Your time before the Lord will refresh your spirit and provide you with a lifeline when it is time to persevere.

My prayer is that with open arms and open hearts, we would prize quiet time with the Lord above all else. The Bible tells us that "he who dwells in the secret place of the Most High shall abide under the shadow of the Almighty" (Psalm 91:1). The secret place. Find that place. Because our strength is found in sitting still in a restless world. Our ceaseless striving is quieted at the foot of the cross.

ACTION STEP

Schedule in time to relax this week rather than overscheduling yourself. A commitment to quiet time is going to bear more fruit than running yourself dry ever will.

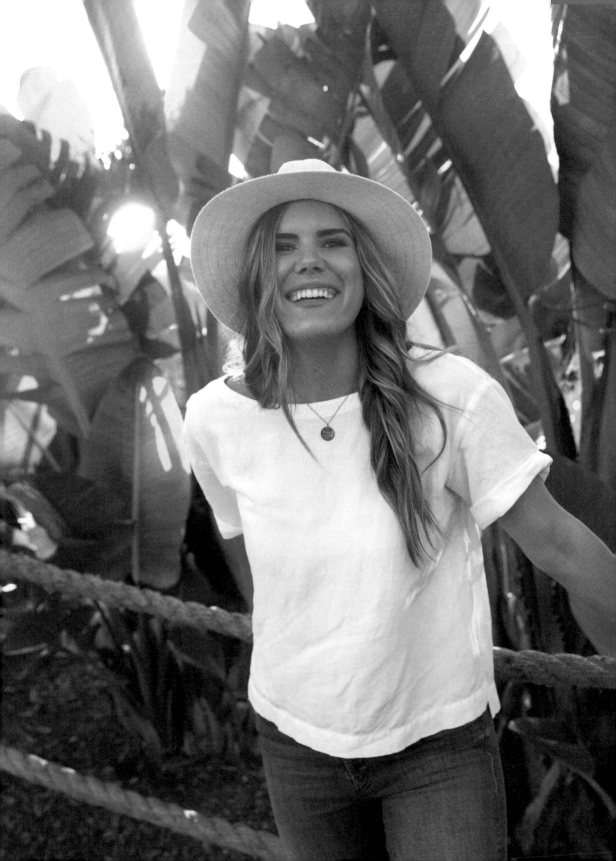

CREATE A REFRESHING MORNING ROUTINE

Gift yourself with a refreshing morning routine to prepare your mind, body, and soul for all that will take place during your waking hours. This is my go-to morning routine. Shape your own ritual to serve your needs.

1. Hydrate before you caffeinate. I say this often because it does wonders to improve energy and digestion.

2. Make your bed. Start your day by tidying your sleep space. This simple act feels productive. At bedtime, you'll be glad to pull back the cover with ease instead of detangling the sheets!

3. Wash your face and nurture your skin. This self-care is invigorating and signals your body to get ready for the new day.

4. Prepare your morning drink with intention. Choose favorite ingredients, brands, and flavors for your tea, coffee, or smoothie so your morning cup is a happy one. Keep tea bags in a pretty container or choose a favorite mug graced with an inspirational saying to brighten your mood.

5. Spend time with God. Read your Bible or a devotional. Write in a prayer or gratitude journal.

6. Get moving. Whether it's a day for a morning workout or not, do something that gets your blood pumping and the oxygen flowing—a short walk, a few jumping jacks, a set of stretches, and so on.

7. Do something unique. Make it routine to do something special each week. Walk to a corner tea shop to get your drink. Go to a farmer's market to buy greens for your smoothie. Take a prayer walk on a new path.

24

JUMP TO
Joy

THIS PAST SUMMER, I had a bad upper-back injury. During my recovery, I couldn't work out for an extended period. I craved my physical routines and the ability to move my body. I missed taking a deep breath without pain too. However, as I lay on the couch one day, I had a lightning-bolt moment of realization: I was different. I was spiritually stronger.

Before God had worked on and in my heart, I would have been upset about missing workouts. My mind would have been preoccupied with worries about ruined progress and setbacks and losing physical ground. I'd be mad. And I likely wouldn't have been able to heal as well or as quickly because of the struggle and misplaced effort. My change of heart showed a God-given strength within me: the newfound strength to choose joy.

Do you have a goal, dream, or plan in your head that nothing and no one is ever going to get in the way of? You will guard it and troubleshoot so there are no disturbances...but then...you didn't see that coming...and just like that, there's a change of plans, a change of landscape.

Obstacles don't get in our way.
They are part of the way.

Can you still choose joy?

Here's what I've learned over the years: Obstacles don't get in our way. They are part of the way. Life is not going to be only open roads with no detours, which is why choosing joy, no matter your circumstance, creates tenacity within you. Jesus did the hardest thing for the joy set before Him. The obstacle of the cross was the way to resurrection, to eternal joy.

Jumping to joy as our response to perceived interruptions or upheavals doesn't always involve choosing the easiest path—it requires that we fix our eyes on the finish line no matter what twists and turns foil our human plans. Following the way of joy invites us to believe that what looks like the end isn't and that something beautiful is continuing to unfold on the horizon.

CHOOSE YOUR REACTION

The strength to endure and the joy to do so come from God. Nehemiah 8:10 says, "Then he said to them, 'Go your way, eat the fat, drink the sweet, and send portions to those for whom nothing is prepared; for this day is holy to our Lord. Do not sorrow, for the joy of the LORD is your strength.'"

The way of moving forward is the way of joy. Let go of frustrations that arise when your path isn't clear. Don't beat yourself up when you fall. Look with new eyes and with God-given strength to view an obstacle as a way toward joy.

We can't predict or control what happens to us, but we can choose how we react: "Count it all joy, my brothers, when you meet trials of various kinds, for you know that the testing of your faith produces steadfastness" (James 1:2–3 ESV).

Commit to the way of joy, friend. It will strengthen you…and it will take you and your dreams amazing places.

If things don't go as planned today, go with the flow and trust in the promise that God will work it for good. Ask Him to specifically show you how to grow from today's wayward path, knowing there is a lesson tucked into today.

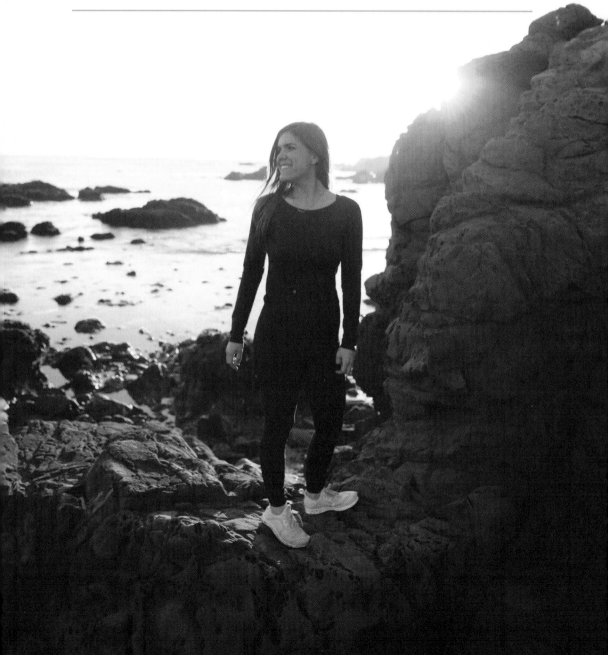

Following the way of joy INVITES US TO BELIEVE THAT WHAT LOOKS LIKE THE END ISN'T AND THAT *something beautiful* IS CONTINUING TO UNFOLD ON THE HORIZON.

25

PREVENT
Burnout

I PICK UP THE PACE OF MY EVENING RUN. It's nearly showtime, and I don't want to miss it. With minutes to spare, I make it to my route's halfway point—a worn, wooden bench, bleached from the salt air. It's here I rest and take in the nightly performance. Born and raised in California, I have a special passion and appreciation for sunsets. As the sun bids farewell to the West Coast, the sky blooms with radiant colors, emitting intensities from pastel to neon. I sigh with awe, certain I have glimpsed heaven.

Maybe that's why I love to run during this time of day so much. I witness God's faithfulness sunset after sunset. He's always there with His luminous artist's palette.

This pause in my workout to take in the view and deep gulps of fresh air was something I refused to allow for years. I believed taking a break midrun would ruin my progress. Not so. I have since learned that I am renewed in body and spirit when I take notice of the world around me and the still small voice within me. We strengthen our bodies, minds, and souls when we make room for rest and refreshment.

God is never in a rush, and He created everything that way, so instead of fighting it, embrace the opportunity to be present in the moment and to be present to your Maker.

How do you prevent burnout? Do you take a beat? Do you allow for a pause? Is there a moment you lift a prayer of thanksgiving for being able to move, run, or simply breathe? Make such spiritual practices a part of your life and even a part of your physical practice, like my run break with a view.

Meditate on Scripture during runs or rounds at the gym. I love using this passage to fix my mind on things above:

> *Those who wait on the LORD shall renew their strength; they shall mount up with wings like eagles, they shall run and not be weary, they shall walk and not faint.*
> ISAIAH 40:31

God is never in a rush, and He created everything that way, so instead of fighting it, embrace the opportunity to be present in the moment and to be present to your Maker.

ACTION STEP

Ask God to help you be content with where you're at today. Ask Him to increase your desire for more of Him rather than for more things that will never satisfy.

CORE CRUSHER

LEVEL: EASY

TIME: 20 MINUTES WITH REST

**ROUTINE: DO EACH EXERCISE FOR 1 MINUTE,
4 SETS, WITH MINIMAL REST BETWEEN SETS**

---

*Bring your A game and crush this core workout! Your core is the foundation
of all movement in the body, so make sure to train your core—it's a must!*

▶️ TURN TO PAGE 221 TO ACCESS VIDEOS FOR THIS WORKOUT!

--- PLANK / V-SITS ---

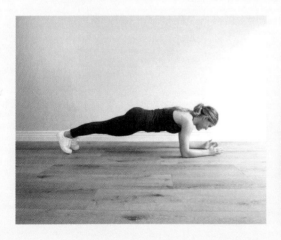 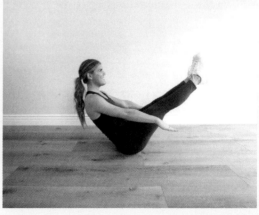

SIDE PLANKS, 30 SECONDS ON EACH SIDE

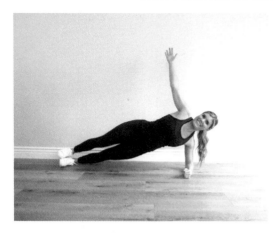
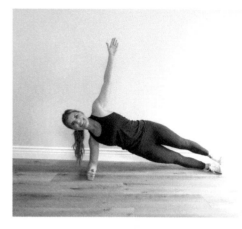

BRIDGES

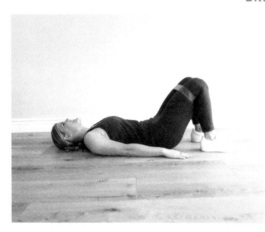
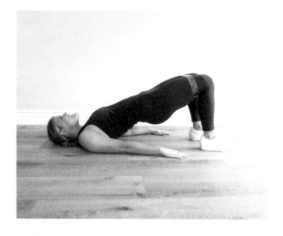

PUSH-UP TO LAT ROWS

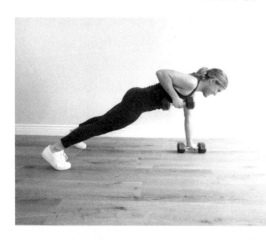
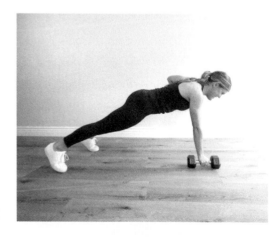

26

REBUILD
THROUGH
Rest

OKAY, THIS IS FOR ANY TYPE A or "gotta finish my checklist" women like me. It might surprise you that the concept of rest was created before the fall of man. So God did not conjure up the concept to give us a break from this sinful world. It is good all by itself. And if God's Word makes a point of mentioning that God Himself rested on the seventh day of the creation process, I'm thinking we have pretty strong motivations to make rest a part of our lives and endeavors. (Let me point out the obvious: Rest was assigned importance long before modern society looked at it as a sign of weakness.)

I used to resist including a rest in my schedule. I'd let guilt ooze into an unscheduled day or afternoon, and before I knew it, I was viewing the idle time as a curse, not a blessing. I saw myself as lazy, unproductive. I'm pretty sure I used terms like

We can do nothing without Jesus,
but we can do all things through Him.

"falling behind" and "wasting time" as my agitation and restlessness increased. It did no good for my body or my soul because I didn't embrace it.

Have you ever felt that way? Are you able to see the value in times of having nothing scheduled, demanded, produced?

God's design for our muscle strengthening and health requires rest. That's right. Our muscles literally need rest and recovery in order to get stronger and keep working! And if we don't get adequate amounts of sleep, our brains and bodies won't function efficiently.

FRUITFUL DOWNTIME

Friend, you and I also need rest and times of stillness to rebuild our spirit and to bear fruit in our lives. What does this look like? Spend time with Jesus, who said,

> *"I am the vine, you are the branches. He who abides in Me, and I in him, bears much fruit."* JOHN 15:5

Only when we're actively abiding in Him will we produce fruit. In our own efforts and striving, we will be fruitless.

John 15:5 closes with Jesus saying, "Without Me, you can do nothing." Yet Philippians 4:13 is true as well: "I can do all things through Christ who strengthens me." Those verses should always go hand in hand. We can do nothing without Jesus, but we can do all things through Him.

The mistake I have made (and can still make) is thinking I can do everything, including taking care of my body, on my own. But trying to do that leads to exhaustion and an unhealthy fear of taking a break.

Our dependence on Christ is going to carry us further than our dependence on ourselves. All too often, we fall short of God's promises by striving instead of abiding in Him peacefully. When you get recharged in your spirit by resting in God and being restored by His truth, you'll move forward like never before...fueled by His eternal strength.

ACTION STEP

Aim for impact before busywork. If everything is important, nothing is. Ask God to direct your steps to do what really matters today.

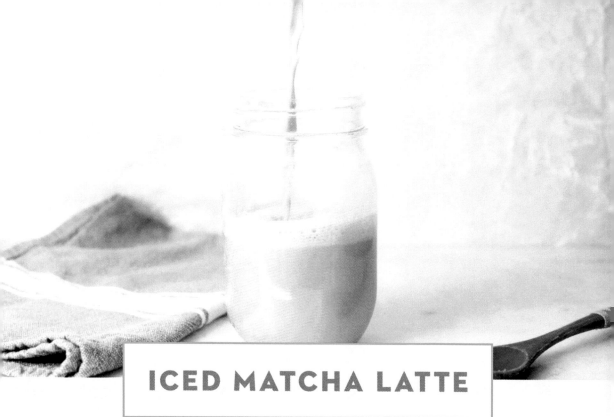

ICED MATCHA LATTE

This refreshing pick-me-up is loaded with antioxidants from the matcha powder. Matcha boosts metabolism and is rich in fiber, chlorophyll, and vitamins. It even aids in concentration! I prefer organic without extra ingredients. You'll find it at any health-food store and some grocery stores.

PREP TIME: **5 MINUTES**   YIELD: **1 SERVING**

---

1 cup Homemade Almond Milk (page 25)
1 tsp. matcha
1 tsp. honey

Blend all the ingredients in a blender.
Pour over ice and enjoy!

HE WILL FIGHT
for You

27

MY CONFESSION OF DEFEAT POURED OUT OF ME one evening after youth group: "I'm going in circles battling my unhealthy eating cycles. I have one good day and then three bad ones. I'm so tired. It feels like I am in a battle without any defenses. It's more like a 24/7 war raging inside me." I was nervous. This wasn't easy. But God was leading me to speak out for help and guidance in the middle of my struggle. I knew this was what I had to do. Even though I told myself I wouldn't cry, the tears started. I looked into the compassion-filled eyes of my youth leader.

She spoke with strength and conviction: "The Lord will fight for you, Cambria. He will fight your battles. Exodus 14:14 says, 'The LORD will fight for you, and you shall hold your peace.'" Like aloe vera on a sunburn, this verse brought relief to my heart and immediately began its healing work. God's Word is a balm that soothes the soul and brings physical refreshment. I was 16 and exhausted. I grabbed ahold of Scripture and God's strength that night.

My part in my healing was to surrender all of me to Christ and then trust Him.

SURRENDER TO WIN

I knew that God was with me and that He was helping me, but what I didn't realize is that God didn't want to just lead the way in this one battle; He wanted to be my Savior and lead the way in all other battles.

It was not my job to beat this eating disorder; it was my job to find rest in Jesus. My part was to surrender to Christ and then trust Him on the path to wellness. That night, I gave up my position as captain and let Jesus step into that rightful role. (It didn't take long to discover that He leads me a lot better than I lead me!)

What can you do when you feel like you keep getting burned? What can you do when you feel like no matter how hard you try, you're getting nowhere? You can choose surrender. You can choose to believe Scripture when it says, "The Lord your God is He who goes with you, to fight for you against your enemies, to save you" (Deuteronomy 20:4).

All those years, I was in a battle for the wrong win. I thought victory would be mine when my outsides matched the ideal I had set for myself and had allowed to become my truth and ruler. There was such relief and joy when I surrendered and let Jesus truly be the King of my life in every single area, including eating and fitness.

When you feel like you're failing, ask God to examine your heart to see if you're fighting the wrong battle. If you are, surrender to Him. That doesn't mean you will never experience missteps again. It means that through Christ, the ultimate victory is yours. Stop fighting and start trusting.

ACTION STEP ─────────────────────────

Keep your Bible next to your nightstand, and leave your phone across the room. When you wake up, instead of reaching for your phone, reach for the life-transforming Scriptures.

─────────────────────────

BACK-2-BACK

LEVEL: MODERATE

TIME: 25 MINUTES WITH REST

ROUTINE: DO EACH EXERCISE FOR 1 MINUTE, 4 SETS

Alternating a basic movement with a high-intensity movement is an effective way to break a sweat and train each muscle group.

▶ TURN TO PAGE 221 TO ACCESS VIDEOS FOR THIS WORKOUT!

SQUATS

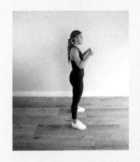
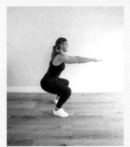
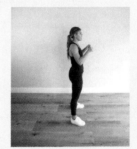
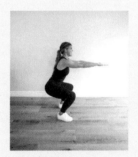

JUMP SQUATS

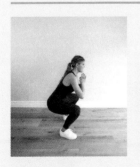
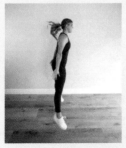
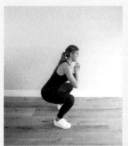
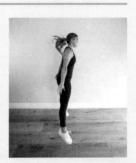

LUNGES

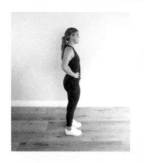 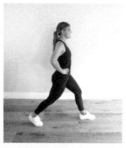 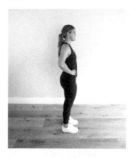 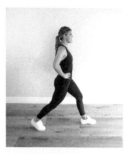

LUNGE JUMPS

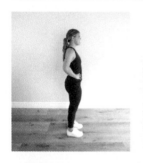 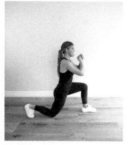 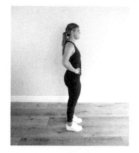 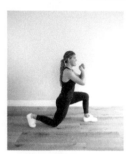

PLANK

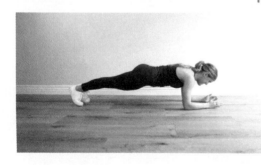 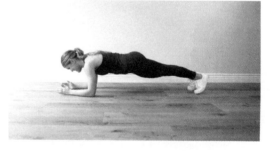

PLANK JACKS

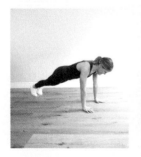 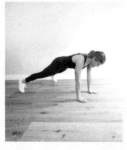 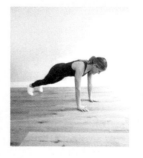 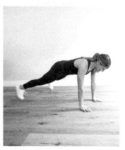

28

MODERATION
Is Strength

THE SMELL OF CHOCOLATE CHIP COOKIES BAKING in the oven is arguably the best smell in the world. Actually, that's not up for debate. It *is* the best smell. The aroma builds our anticipation for those warm, delicious, gooey treats. But what if you just got back from the gym where you gave it your all? You're tired, you're hungry, and those cookies smell amazing, but you don't want to negate that killer workout, right?

What to do, what to do?

First, let me make it clear that there's nothing wrong with eating a cookie. I don't care what a diet says, you can eat that cookie and enjoy every bite, free of guilt. But if you're anything like me and have struggled with food and body image, you know it might not be that simple.

When God was leading me down the path of healing, I wasn't able to stop at only one cookie. Or two. Once I started, I kept on going until I was bingeing. Believe me,

I don't care what a diet says, you can eat that cookie and enjoy every bite, free of guilt.

there is no pleasure in this experience. First Peter 2:11 says, "Beloved, I beg you as sojourners and pilgrims, abstain from fleshly lusts which war against the soul." My eating disorder and habits were about much more than satisfying hunger. When someone binge eats, they don't taste food or delight in it. It isn't the same as enjoying a few pieces of a deep-dish pie with extra cheese on Friday night. I was in bondage and had no self-control.

Therefore, before I could enjoy cookies in moderation without overeating, I knew I had to develop a healthy relationship with food again. I gave up sugary food. This was not a new diet; it was a way for me to physically deny my flesh so that I might be free from it. In no way was this a new diet or food restriction. This didn't have to do with the physical but rather was about the spiritual.

I didn't decide to permanently give up sugar and treats. Instead, after careful consideration, I chose to abstain from sugar for a period of time. I eat cookies now and enjoy them; it's wonderful, delicious, and freeing all at the same time. I continue to lean into God's strength to heal my relationship with food, and He so faithfully has.

PUT DOWN THE WEIGHTS

What weighs you down or works against your pursuit of true health and balanced living? For you, it might not be about food at all. Maybe it is your perspective about exercise. Maybe you stay up all night viewing social media and you deprive your body of necessary sleep. You might work too much and too often and rarely take time for family or friends or God. Whatever you use in excess to fill an inner void needs to be replaced with God, His love, and His grace.

Eating cookies is not a sin. But obsessing about food and idolizing my appearance was. In the past, I binged on sweets when I hadn't had enough food during the day.

Both of those actions are offtrack for honoring my body as a temple. Breaking the cycle of restrictive eating helped me then shed the burden of binge eating.

Practicing moderation is a strength. And it requires effort and building up to it. It takes recognizing the things that are weighing you down so you can make changes. Whatever your area of "too much" may be, remember that the Bible says in Hebrews 12:1, "Let us lay aside every weight, and the sin which so easily ensnares us, and let us run with endurance the race that is set before us." What an invitation! Laying aside our burdens allows us to be free to run with ease and joy toward all that God has for us tomorrow.

ACTION STEP

Grace before guilt. Next time you're tempted to fall into the trap of guilt, ask God to help you overcome these destructive thoughts by His power.

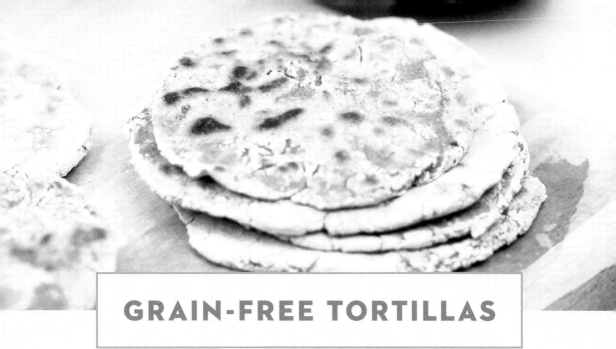

GRAIN-FREE TORTILLAS

These tortillas are my obsession! They are the perfect combination of thick and chewy but firm. They're filling and satisfying—a perfect snack on their own or when used for a wrap.

PREP TIME: 20 MINUTES   YIELD: 8 SERVINGS

---

1 cup blanched almond flour
1¾ cups arrowroot flour
(plus extra for rolling the dough)
1 tsp. xanthan gum

Pinch of salt
½ cup warm water
2 T. honey

In a mixer, combine and blend the dry ingredients. Slowly add the water and honey. Sprinkle a clean surface with some extra arrowroot flour, and roll out the well-mixed dough into the preferred size and shape. Cook directly over medium heat in a sauté pan. Serve immediately with your favorite toppings, such as salsa, avocado, grilled chicken or tofu, black beans, melted cheese, or grilled veggies. These are also delicious with almond butter and jam or honey.

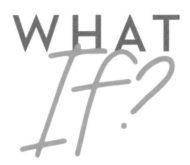

29

WHAT If?

A LOT OF US HAVE THIS IDEA OF WHAT HEALTHY looks like: waking up early, drinking lemon water, completing an early workout, drinking a green smoothie postworkout, going about the day downing lots of water, and returning home at five to do a second, similar routine in the evening.

But what if there's something deeper here? Indulge me for a moment as you read through this list of what-ifs; see if something stands out as possible, as true for your life:

- What if the simple idea of a healthy life has gotten a lot more complex than it ought to be?
- What if being healthy isn't just about getting in a jog and sipping on vitamin-rich juice?
- What if it's not about constantly trying to improve your appearance?

When we let God into every area of
our lives, they all get less complicated.
We find balance and rhythms of grace.

- What if beauty is facing yourself and embracing yourself?
- What if relaxing and eating brownies on the couch sometimes is just as healthy as being disciplined and focused in the gym?
- What if it's daring to see past the physical and brave to look inside?
- What if enjoying a hot chocolate is as healthy as sipping lemon-infused water?
- What if looking in the mirror and accepting every part of yourself is as healthy as looking in the mirror and wanting to get stronger? (What if you did both at the same time?)
- What if you evaluated your heart as often as you evaluate yourself in the mirror?
- What if standing on your identity in Christ is far healthier than standing on a scale?
- What if strength and motivation came from words of truth instead of words of criticism?

When we let God into every area of our lives, they all get less complicated. We find balance and rhythms of grace. A healthy perspective shift can do wonders for our outlook on life. Try it this morning and see how it influences your day.

ACTION STEP
Evaluate your heart today and not your image in the mirror.

FULL-BODY SCULPT

LEVEL: **MODERATE**

TIME: **25 MINUTES WITH REST**

ROUTINE: **4 SETS**

---

*Get ready to get fit from head to toe. This simple
sculpting workout will have you sweating and smiling.*

▶ TURN TO PAGE 221 TO ACCESS VIDEOS FOR THIS WORKOUT!

—— **1-MINUTE PLANK** ——

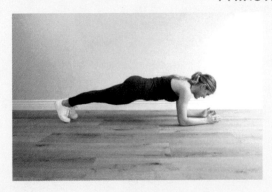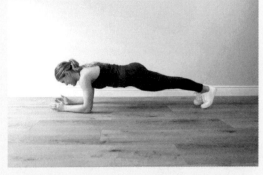

10 BURPEES

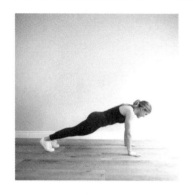 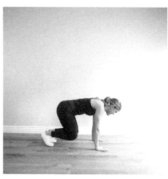 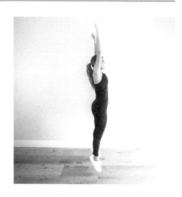

12 REVERSE LUNGES

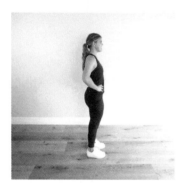 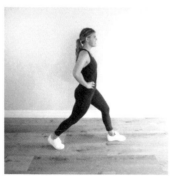 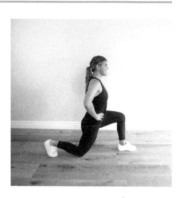

10 TRICEP PUSH-UPS

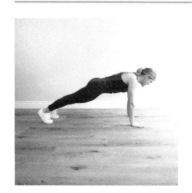 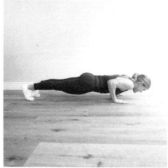 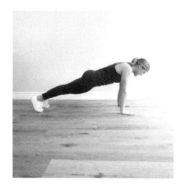

30

PRESS ON AND
Press In

BEING FIT AND GROWING IN STRENGTH bring some bittersweet moments. Do you happen to know this one? You're happy that you're getting stronger and yet in pain from a gym session. If you've ever tried sitting down after an intense leg workout, you know what I'm talking about! If you hike to the top of a crest, it's so challenging that you might want to quit halfway because your lower back is rebelling, but you press on. It's all worth it when you look at that view! Personally, I must regularly remind myself that sore today means strong tomorrow.

I love those physical and spiritual mountaintop experiences; it's refreshing up there. But our endurance is not built on the actual mountain top; it is tested and developed on our way up. We might be inspired on the apex, but the fruit, the substance, is grown in the depths of the valley.

> When we want to give up, that is when
> we need to lift up our cares to God.

GOD IS IN THE VALLEY

When we want to give up, that is when we need to lift up our cares to God and trust that "all things work together for good to those who love God, to those who are the called according to His purpose" (Romans 8:28). We grow to where we need to go.

God didn't lead me down my personal valley. I led myself there when I thought I knew what I was doing. But you can bet He was in the valley with me. God is so merciful and loving that He brought good out of what was bad. He was growing me despite my mistakes.

Even in the lowest parts of life, God will grow you for your own good. Don't give up. Press on and press in because you will reap a harvest if you do not give up (Galatians 6:9). If your trial is to stay committed to healthy choices, God cares. If your valley experience has to do with making ends meet or repairing a broken relationship, God is in it with you. You will feel the ache of learning patience and how to endure with faith even as God is moving within your willing spirit and your situation. No matter what your daily struggle is, it can all come together for good.

Ask God to help you see His redemptive power in your circumstances.

ACTION STEP

Next time you feel like you failed during or after a workout, proclaim a scriptural truth over it.

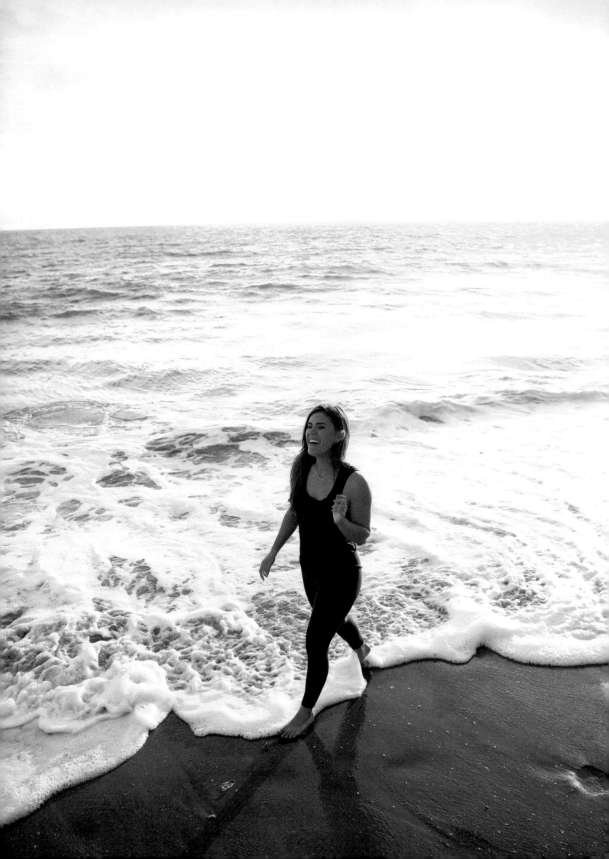

WALK FOR JOY AND FITNESS

Celebrate your commitment to moving as you make your way along wooded paths or city sidewalks toward better health. There are so many benefits. Here are some simple ways to make the most of your walks:

1. Use shoes that offer you the level of support your feet and body need. Many good shoe stores will evaluate your gait to help you choose the best option.

2. Start your walk with a slow pace to warm up, a slightly faster pace to get your heart rate up, and then a cooldown tempo to help your muscles recover.

3. If you want to track your walks, an app or device can provide information and motivation. But those extras aren't necessary! Every ten days, add 5 minutes or a third of a mile to your routine. After one month, you'll be walking 15 minutes or one mile further. It adds up.

4. Create a motivating playlist or select podcasts or audiobooks to listen to. If you save the next episode or chapter until the next workout, you'll be motivated to get back to it!

5. Bring a friend or start a walking group. What is more fun than being able to get healthy and strong while getting to know others better?

6. Memorize a verse or inspirational quote to think about during your walk. Or use your walk as a time to pray for others. This gives your times of moving even more meaning for your life and health.

31

BEAUTY IS
Soul Deep

LET'S BE REAL. I want to be confident with myself, and I know you do too. So how do we find inner peace with our outer selves?

I wrestled with this for a long time. Here's what God's Word revealed: "Do not let your adornment be merely outward—arranging the hair, wearing gold, or putting on fine apparel—rather let it be the hidden person of the heart, with the incorruptible beauty of a gentle and quiet spirit, which is very precious in the sight of God" (1 Peter 3:3-4).

If there's an incorruptible beauty, then there's also a corruptible beauty. When we focus merely on what's outward, like the verse says, we are focusing on improving our corruptible beauty. There's nothing wrong with a pretty face—and don't get me wrong, I do love my squats and my makeup—but there's something deeper here. A

A beautiful face cannot compare
with a beautiful heart.

beautiful face cannot compare with a beautiful heart. Jesus is talking about an eternal beauty here that has nothing to do with fixing our hair or wearing cute clothes.

The real beauty that is incorruptible and eternal is found only in the heart. When we spend more time or only place importance on our outward self instead of developing a gentle and quiet spirit, we're not going to attain real, true beauty. It's not going to last. Some of the most beautiful women I've ever met have gray hair and plenty of wisdom-made wrinkles.

What a vessel holds is more important than the vessel itself. Look at it this way: I'd rather drink a delicious beverage out of an ugly mug than sip expired milk in fine china. I bet you would too. The apostle Peter is right: Don't let your adornment merely be outward. If it's more important to you to make it to the gym than it is to meet with Jesus, it's time to reevaluate your standard of beauty. How much time do you spend on your inward beauty in comparison to your outward appearance? Do you feel like it could use some balancing?

Ask God to help you place importance on your inner beauty. Make a habit of reading your Bible and talking to the Lord daily, just like you regularly wake up, get dressed, and put on your makeup. Make spending time with Jesus part of your beauty routine.

ACTION STEP

Find your passion before following the crowd. Instead of following the latest fitness fad, follow what's on your heart. What's your favorite way to move? Now do it!

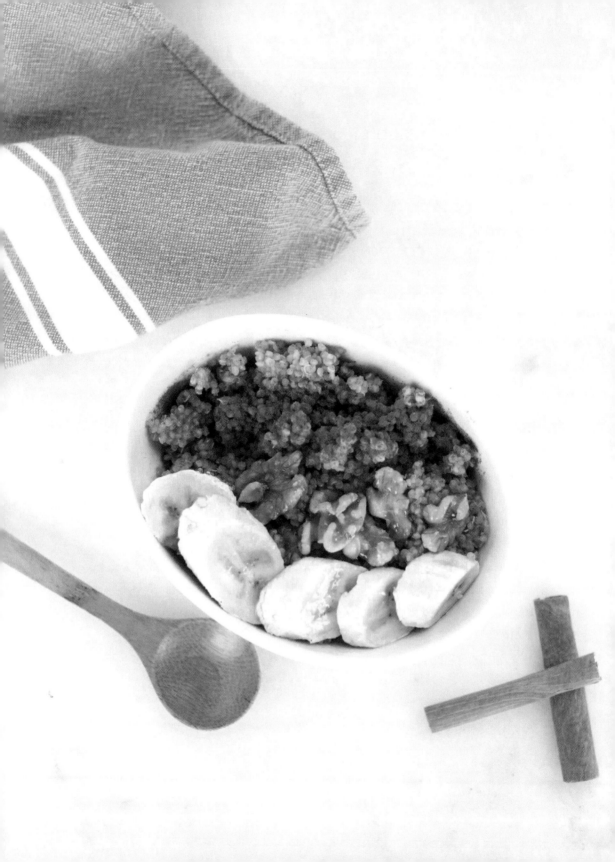

BREAKFAST QUINOA

*Yes—quinoa for breakfast! I promise, it is the creamiest,
tastiest, heartiest way to start your day.
This warm meal is packed with protein and fiber.*

PREP TIME: **20 MINUTES**   YIELD: **1 SERVING**

---

1 cup water

1 cup quinoa

¼ cup almond milk

½ mashed banana

¼ tsp. cinnamon

1 tsp. honey

Add water and the quinoa to a saucepan and bring to a boil. Once
boiling, reduce to low heat and cover with a lid for 15 minutes until
done. Mix in the almond milk and mashed banana. Once well combined
and heated through, sprinkle with cinnamon and drizzle with honey.
Get creative with toppings—add more banana, nuts, or granola.

32

INSIDE-OUT
Strength

AS I MENTIONED IN THIS SECTION'S OPENING STORY, my trainer, Jan, is special to me. She's been my trainer ever since I started working out at age 15 and since I started my YouTube channel! About a year ago, I had my final sweat session with her, and it gave me a chance to reflect on her impact on my life.

My answer surprised even me: She changed my heart.

Yes, she challenged my physical limits in every workout. She made working out fun. She taught me how to push through discomfort and embrace the strength that comes through persevering.

But even more importantly, God used her to teach me about becoming the strongest version of myself *inside*. Interestingly, her emotional and spiritual training occurred through what she didn't say and didn't do.

Jan is shredded, tan, and incredibly fit. But she never talked about it. She was my trainer when I was struggling with binge eating, and not once did she remark about my body. She didn't praise me for finally getting more toned or point out when I was gaining weight. She modeled strength from the inside out through what she emphasized, held with value, and built up in others.

I admire her because her passion for loving and serving others with kindness and wisdom—the fruit of her faith—is evident. Her inner strength took the lead.

That's why 1 Timothy 4:8 says physical training is of some value instead of saying it holds the utmost value. The verse goes on to say that godliness has value for all things, holding promise for both the present life and the life to come. So what is physical training missing?

The life to come.

I'm sharing this because I want you to become the strongest version of yourself. What does that mean? It includes...

- recognizing that true strength is found not externally but internally,
- being grounded in truth,
- thinking first of your spirit when you look at yourself,
- wholeheartedly embracing who God says you are instead another's idea of you,
- living a life filled with grace rather than perfection, and
- resting and laughing and being able to eat cookies *and* salads with joy.

How do you and I become women who are strong inside and out? We shift to an eternal mindset! We work out to become transformed from within so that the evidence of our faith serves Christ, our purpose in Him, and the people He places along our journey.

The world knows when they encounter an inside-and-out strong woman...not because they "feel the burn" but because they feel the love.

ACTION STEP

Choose quiet thoughts tonight instead of TV. Turn off Netflix and let your thoughts flow onto the blank pages of a journal so they aren't swimming around your mind.

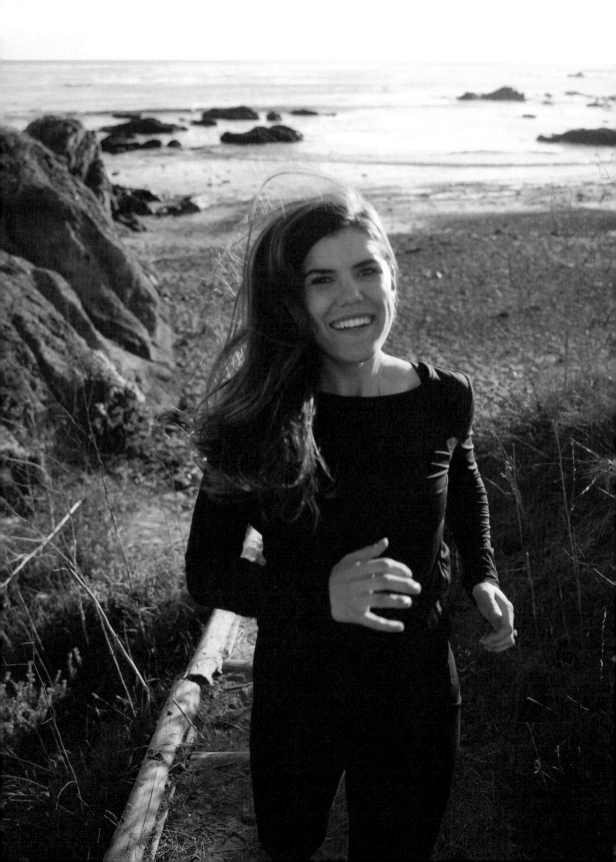

MOMENTUM WITH A HEART-RATE MONITOR

If you know me, you know I don't like to emphasize numbers in the fitness journey. So this might shock you...I love heart-rate monitors.

Some days I wear the monitor during my workout to motivate myself to become stronger. Other days I wear my heart-rate monitor because it's a physical reminder of the energy I'm investing. Think of it as an optional way to fuel your workout with information and motivation.

Our heart rate lets us know our level of effort. Here is the basic formula to calculate your maximum heart rate:

220 - your age = your MHR

There are fancier ways to calculate your MHR, but this gets you started. Before you push toward any range, talk with your doctor because we all have other factors that can impact our health.

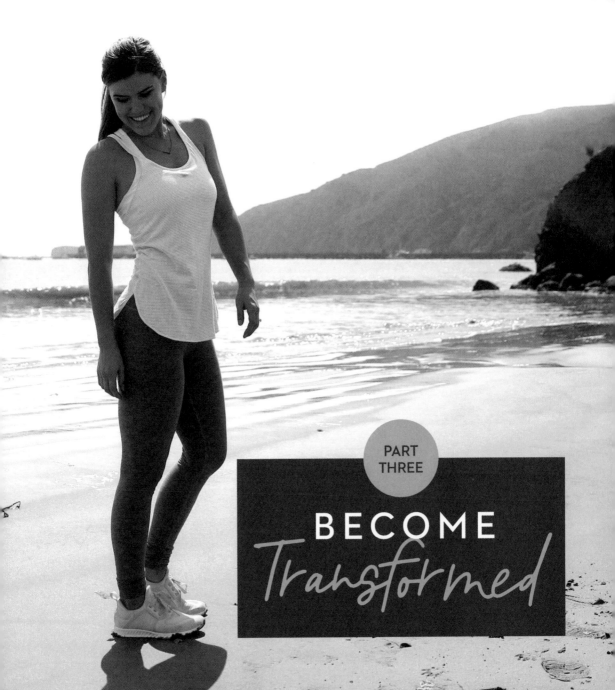

PART
THREE

BECOME
Transformed

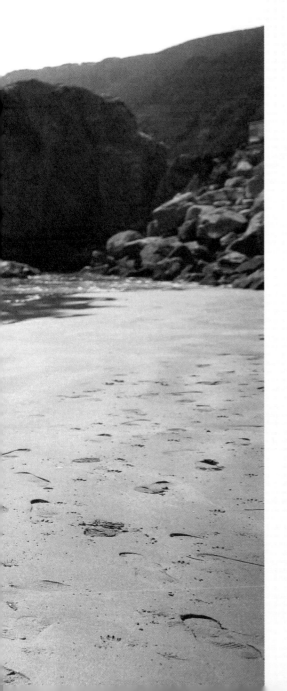

I put on my running shoes and head to the kitchen to prep the snacks I'll showcase on my YouTube vlog episode today. I'm eager to share a few simple ways to make healthy choices with my subscribers and others. My husband, Bo, and I joke around as he gets the camera ready and I chop (and eat) a few strawberries. The ritual of preparing food often leads me to pray. Today, my eyes are fixed on the brilliant red of this nutritious food, and my heart is fixed on the brilliant joy of this healthy life.

I pause to appreciate this moment. God is so faithful. He has guided me to become motivated, strong, and transformed in my physical and spiritual life. I am a changed Cambria. And I am the person God created me to be from the very beginning.

Lately, I've faced quite a few transitions and tough days with many unknowns. A few years ago, such uncertainty would have derailed my healthy choices and my emotions. But today, all I feel is gratitude, peace, and a sense of being cared for by God. I'm hopeful and ready to embrace whatever He has planned for me.

I hope you're starting to feel changes within. Together, let's continue this journey with anticipation for the great things to come. God is shaping us into strong women who trust Him.

33

IDENTITY
makeover

HOW DO YOU OVERCOME INSECURITY? By standing firm in your God-given identity. Notice I didn't say your self-made identity. We are much more than what we think and say about ourselves; in fact, most of our insecurity is born in our self-evaluation. We believe we're not enough so we live as if that's true. We try harder to become better, prettier, more beautiful, but eventually, burnout and comparison eat away at us.

Do you experience insecurity? Do you want to be secure in your God-given identity and learn to live in the light of what God says about you? Are you tired of comparing yourself to anyone or everyone? Are you exhausted trying to measure up to your own standard?

Our security comes from knowing who we are, and that begins by knowing who we're not. You aren't created to perfect your image. You're not who you feel you are on

Our security comes from knowing who we are, and that begins by knowing who we're not. You aren't created to perfect your image.

those rough days. You need a firmer foundation to grow and become who God made you to be. That foundation is your security in Christ.

By now you know I'm not the girl who has it all together. I'm the girl who found rest in my weakness because that's where God is strong on my behalf. I'm the girl who realized trying to live up to a self-made identity was crazy-making and unrelenting. The false story of who I was had led me to a place of brokenness and discouragement. I'm the girl who needed God for all things.

GLORY IS IN THE STORY

My hope for you is that you'll see the goodness of God in your big struggles or daily obstacles. The trials you face are forging in you a warrior-like spirit. My pastor, Jon Courson, once told me that everybody wants the testimony without the test. But the test you're going through is the part of your story that ultimately brings God glory. There can be peace and joy in the persevering because you know you are being shaped and molded into a new creation.

You and I know this mindset from the work and effort of exercise. We are reshaping and becoming transformed, and it wouldn't happen without those moments of difficulty and sweat. Those are the times we push through and use as a catalyst to keep going. As we recount to others our stories of physical and spiritual transformation, we will also speak of the joy.

Before I understood I needed to surrender all things to God, I obsessed over the shape of my body. And then one day, I encountered a profound truth in a deeper way:

The search will cease at the cross.

Jesus's body was broken for me. Of course, I would surrender my own body to the Savior. That's the day I was set free.

What we're all searching for is Jesus, whether we try to find Him in being skinny or in happiness or fitness. Whatever it is that we're looking for, it's found in Him. Our identity makeovers happen when we overcome the ideals we set as idols. And that only happens in Christ.

For some of us, the quest takes us along some crazy paths. For others, it is filled with many questions and missteps. And still others will find it rife with battles of the spirit. But for all of us, the search will cease at the cross.

ACTION STEP

Write down two goals for your physical makeover and your spiritual makeover. Have them grounded in joy and not perfection.

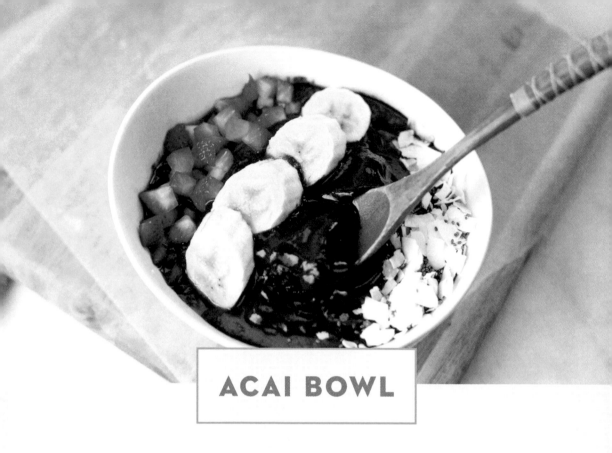

ACAI BOWL

A refreshing acai bowl packs an antioxidant punch filled with vitamins and fiber that leave you full and satisfied. This bowl is sure to make your taste buds smile.

PREP TIME: **5 MINUTES**   YIELD: **1 SERVING**

1 acai packet
1 frozen banana
1 cup frozen blueberries

¼ cup frozen mango
¼ cup frozen strawberries
½ cup almond milk

Add the fruit to a blender and slowly add almond milk until it's the desired consistency. Less liquid equals a thicker bowl. Top with extras, like freshly chopped fruit and Grain-Free Granola (page 81)!

34

CLAIM YOUR
Capability

I'VE ENCOURAGED YOU TO NOT FOCUS on the mirror when you're investing in a long-term healthy lifestyle. However, today I want you to. How about right now? Take this with you and go stand in front of the nearest mirror.

Take a breath. Let it out. Do it again.

Follow along with me by saying to your reflection, "I don't want or need to change anything to feel fully loved and accepted. I desire only to be changed from the inside out."

How does that feel? Are you being honest? Are you still in the process of believing this? It takes great strength to look in the mirror and not want to change one thing. Why? Because by this point in our lives, we are programmed to do that. We also look for aspects of other people we think should be changed. Many of us do this as a default action or reaction. That's something we can change in this journey.

Do a joy-giving workout because you love the body God designed and you want to take care of it.

I know that you're strong, and I want you to start walking in that strength.

Let go of that first response and reprogram your heart and mind so that you see what God sees in you and in others. This creates quite a shift in our relationships and perspectives.

Now look at your reflection and say, "I am capable and strong in the Lord. God's power will shape my heart, body, and soul for His purpose."

From here on out, every time you look in the mirror or go work out, I want you to remember you can choose to love yourself and your workout. You don't need to do a dreadful weights or cardio set because you're unhappy with the way you look. Do a joy-giving workout because you love the body God designed and you want to take care of it.

See the difference? A small change in mentality can change your whole world.

YOU BELONG TO GOD

As a masterpiece created by God, you are capable in His ability. You're strong. You're confident. You're restored. You're redeemed. You're renewed. Claim those as your truths. You only have one life, one today, one body, and this moment. Why not enjoy taking care of it and doing what you love?

The shift from crafting my perfect body to simply honoring God with my body no matter how it looks changed my outlook. First Corinthians 6:19 says,

> *Don't you know that your body is the temple of the Holy Spirit, who lives in you and who was given to you by God? You do not belong to yourselves but to God.*

If I am created by God, belong to God, and want to live for God, then everything that I do can either glorify Him or glorify myself. First Corinthians 6:20 says, "You were bought at a price. Therefore glorify God with your body."

These shifts are already happening. You've invested in this journey to become healthy in your body and soul. Accept your God-given body and commit to taking care of it because it's a gift. This week, exercise in a way that's enjoyable for you and glorifying to Him. You can do this!

ACTION STEP

Today, stop eating when you feel satisfied. Enjoy knowing you can save that last bite for later by honoring your hunger cues when you're full.

AS A MASTERPIECE CREATED BY GOD,
YOU ARE CAPABLE IN HIS ABILITY.

You're strong. You're confident. You're restored.
You're redeemed. You're renewed.

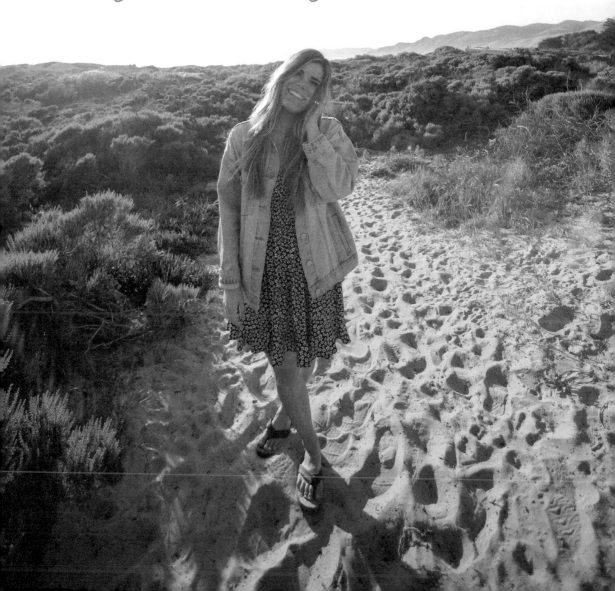

35

BUILD ON
A SOLID
Foundation

WHILE YOU WALK AROUND THE PARK EACH WEEK or incorporate stretches into your morning routine, you might not be thinking about how each movement can honor God. Yet this is the gift of the believer's life. What we do with our time, minds, and bodies can honor Jesus: "Whatever you do, do it heartily, as to the Lord and not to men, knowing that from the Lord you will receive the reward of the inheritance; for you serve the Lord Christ" (Colossians 3:23-24).

Give your all to your call to walk on a path of healing and health. Tell others who you are honoring by caring for your body and spirit. Inspire and support your journey to becoming fit with verses that encourage your heart.

When I first started working out, I didn't ever think about honoring God with my body. I simply cared about what my body looked like. If I'm being honest, pride motivated my first efforts toward fitness. However, I learned through reading Matthew 7:24-26 that we can lay the right foundation for every action in our lives.

What we do with our time, minds, and bodies can honor Jesus.

"Whoever hears these sayings of Mine, and does them, I will liken him to a wise man who built his house on the rock: and the rain descended, the floods came, and the winds blew and beat on that house; and it did not fall, for it was founded on the rock. But everyone who hears these sayings of Mine, and does not do them, will be like a foolish man who built his house on the sand." MATTHEW 7:24–26

When our actions come from a heart with good intentions that are rooted in God's Word, we lay the right foundation for everything that we do with our lives.

How many times have you attempted to do something, but your plans fell through—or maybe you gave up too quickly because discouragement got the best of you? When it comes to living healthy, a foundation that honors our God-given bodies is what we need. If we have an eternal mindset in everything we do, our foundation will be sure.

WALK ON THE BEACH, BUT DON'T BUILD THERE

When Christ became my foundation for all things, my desire to work out increased because I wasn't focused on my performance. I just kept my eyes on Jesus, and when the discouragement, comparison, worry, or self-pity tried to knock me out, my house did not fall. In fact, because I had weathered the storm, my confidence in Christ actually increased. He is our rock. Instead of building our plans on the sand, we can build our whole lives and everything that we do on the rock of Jesus, knowing that He is a firm foundation.

The Bible says, "You are worthy, O Lord, to receive glory and honor and power; for You created all things, and by Your will they exist and were created" (Revelation 4:11). We are created for God's pleasure. How amazing that we can honor and please the Lord as we enjoy getting healthy. All the more reason to celebrate this part of your life and never turn it into drudgery.

Has anyone in your life noticed your transformation? Is there evidence in your attitude and confidence that you are building a life on a solid foundation? If someone asks you how or why your physical health and attitude have improved, you can answer, "I'm serving and pleasing the Lord!"

ACTION STEP

Take a look at your fitness goal and then measure your progress based on the steps you've taken to reach your goal rather than how far you have to go to get there.

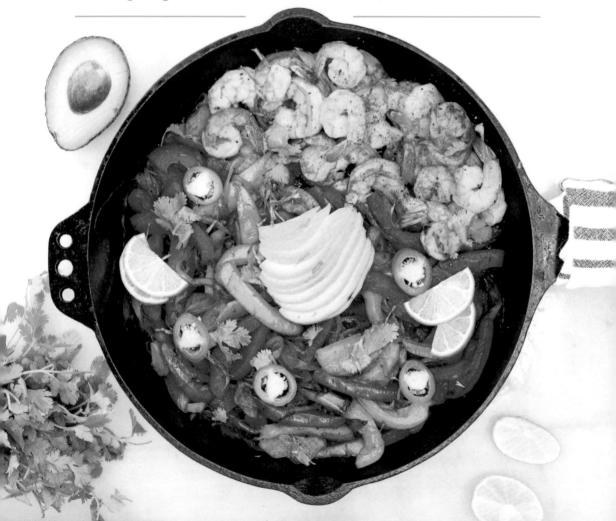

SHEET-PAN FAJITAS

One of my favorite go-to meals is a tray dinner or a sheet-pan dinner.
It's quick, easy to clean up, and provides a full and complete meal!

PREP TIME: 25 MINUTES   YIELD: 4 SERVINGS

---

1 T. chili powder
Salt and pepper to taste
3 large bell peppers
1 large sweet onion
2 T. avocado oil
Protein of choice (I like chicken or shrimp with this recipe)
Juice of 1 lime
Grain-Free Tortillas (page 133)
Guacamole, hot sauce, salsa, and lime wedges for serving

Preheat your broiler to high. Combine the chili powder, salt, and pepper into a small bowl. Slice the peppers and onions and put them on the baking sheet, drizzle with 1 tablespoon of the avocado oil, and season with half the seasoning mixture. Broil until softened and starting to char (about 10 minutes). Add the uncooked protein, either chicken or shrimp, on top of the peppers, drizzle with the other tablespoon of avocado oil, and sprinkle the remaining seasoning over the top. Return the baking sheet to the broiler until protein is cooked through (about 5 or 10 minutes). Drizzle with the lime juice and serve with warmed tortillas, guacamole, hot sauce, salsa, and lime wedges. Enjoy!

36

FOLLOW
THE
Leader

HAVE YOU EVER STUMBLED OUT OF BED EARLY, gotten dressed, headed off to live your day, and the realized at two in the afternoon that your shirt is inside-out? This is what I did years ago…except the thing that was inside-out wasn't my favorite top. It was my view of healthy living.

My version of being healthy was to avoid cupcakes like the plague and put in a lot of exercise hours. Here's the simple truth, because I need to be reminded of it myself: God looks at the heart. And it is the condition of our spiritual heart that measures our health, well-being, and wholeness.

We can open up the Bible and see mention after mention of the importance of what is inside a person. Even the description of Jesus doesn't focus on the outward man:

There was nothing beautiful or majestic about his appearance, nothing to attract us to him. ISAIAH 53:2 NLT

> It is the condition of our spiritual heart that measures our health, well-being, and wholeness.

A FAITH OF NO FAVORITES

The book of James explores the importance of not showing favoritism to people based on their appearance or status. If a rich man walks into church dressed nicely compared to the poor man who comes in filthy, we are not to vary the way we welcome each person. Jesus shows no favoritism. He loved the whole world and whoever believes in Him will be saved.

When David was anointed to be king, he wasn't picked because of his good looks. In fact, he almost wasn't picked at all because of how small he was! When the prophet Samuel came to anoint one of Jesse's sons, Jesse didn't even bother to go get David. Surely the shepherd boy should go about tending his sheep, not tending a kingdom. But God spoke through His prophet Samuel and declared that the Lord doesn't look at one's outward appearance; He looks at the heart.

My friend, this ancient truth is still true in our modern world today. God's looking for a heart that's after Him. Let this truth about the spiritual heart also transform your efforts to strengthen your physical one.

ACTION STEP

Start your day by reading a psalm and adding a tablespoon of MCT oil to your coffee or tea for an extra energy boost.

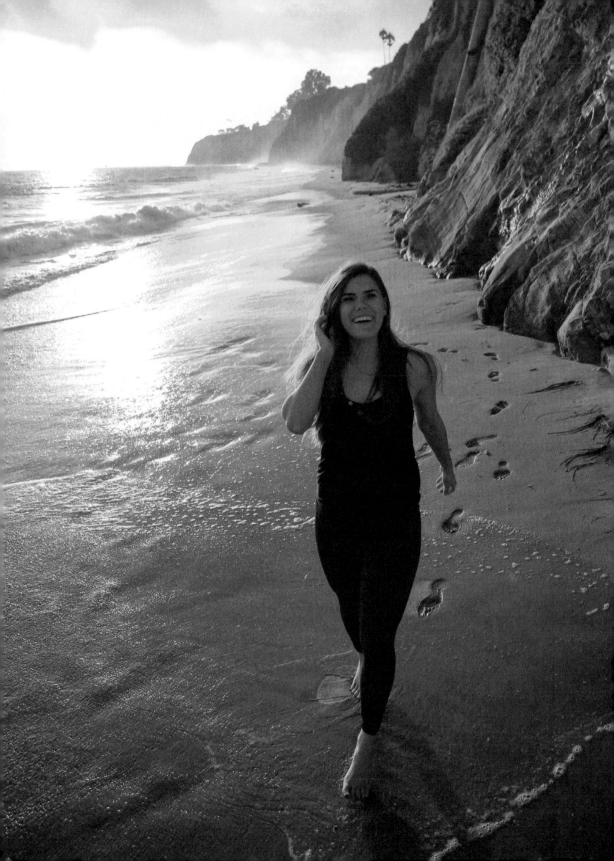

DESIGN A STRESS-REDUCING NIGHTLY ROUTINE

In this journey to becoming you and becoming strong, sleep will be your friend. Map out some basic steps that will gently nudge you to slow down, breathe deeply, and prepare for quality sleep.

1. **Take care of what matters most.** Plan early in the day to finish the important things on your to-do list so you can ease into your evening with more joy and less stress.

2. **Use a scent to let your body know it's time to wind down.** You could use a scented spray, a candle, or an essential-oil diffuser. I use lavender and ylang-ylang oil in my diffuser. The moment I take in those scents, my body relaxes. Here's one of my favorite tricks: I put those two oils and some carrier oil in a roller bottle and rub the mixture on the bottom of my feet right before I go to sleep. Ahhh.

3. **Start winding down at the same time each evening.** Try for an hour or two before bed. It helps so much! The first action could be to step away from technology. Shift to reading books or magazines or spending time journaling, drawing, or coloring.

4. **Sip on a healthy, stress-reducing drink.** I love to make Golden Mylk (page 187) or a nighttime tea with chamomile and mint. Drink from a favorite mug.

5. **Create a self-care routine for bedtime.** Try a facial mask or a leisurely bath by candlelight. Enjoy a mellow form of movement: a relaxed swim, easy stretches, or a gentle yoga routine.

CHANGED
AND
Unchained

WE CAN BE SET FREE FROM OUR CIRCUMSTANCES. We can have joy inside us no matter what's going on around us. How do we experience freedom like that? How do we have joy inside us when everything seems to be going wrong around us? Let's take a look at this story in Acts to hear a firsthand account of what real freedom is:

> *At midnight Paul and Silas were praying and singing hymns to God, and the prisoners were listening to them. Suddenly there was a great earthquake, so that the foundations of the prison were shaken; and immediately all the doors were opened and everyone's chains were loosed. And the keeper of the prison, awaking from sleep and seeing the prison doors open, supposing the prisoners had fled, drew his sword and was about to kill himself. But Paul called with a loud voice, saying, "Do yourself no harm, for we are all here."* ACTS 16:25–28

May you be known for living out your liberty
in Christ with such joy and passion that
other hearts see the way to lasting freedom
and are changed from within.

Paul and Silas were in prison because in the name of Jesus, they had cast out a spirit from a fortune-telling girl. This girl was a slave who had been making money for her masters. When those masters heard of what had been done, they were angry. Their source of profit had just gone down the drain. So they dragged Paul and Silas to the authorities, who beat them and threw them in jail. How. Insane. Is. That?

They had their backs beaten brutally and then were thrown into the depths of prison. Don't you think they had a reason to be upset? Isn't that unfair? Yet what do Paul and Silas do? They start not only praying but singing out loud to God. And the other prisoners were listening in. When the prison doors were closed, they had a freedom so deep that they praised God. When the prison doors were opened, they didn't try to run away into freedom because they were already free. (There's that "what's inside is what matters" theme again.)

SOUL FREEDOM

Paul and Silas didn't praise God when He set them free. First they praised God, and then they were set free. There's a big difference between those. They were already free deep down in their souls. After the prison door incident, the keeper of the prison was fearful everyone had fled and was ready to kill himself, but Paul stopped him and cried out, "We are all here." Isn't that amazing? Paul and Silas stayed. And the other prisoners didn't exit either; instead, they looked in amazement at Paul and Silas. How strange and fascinating these two were. Here they were in jail, singing songs to God.

They didn't run when the way was clear, and they basically saved the prison keeper from death. Their soul-deep freedom was radical and influenced the choices and lives of those around them.

You and I can do and be the same. Our soul-deep freedom changes us and changes our interactions with others. We are no longer confined by people. And we don't confine them to prisons of shame either. We build up those around us because we aren't comparing or becoming envious. We definitely don't need to keep checking the scale, because it's no longer our prison or our key to freedom. We're free, my friend. Free to live in a profound, transformed way that might stun folks around us.

When we're in troubled circumstances that may be viewed as chains by the world, people are watching. People are watching us and what we choose to do. Knowing this, what will we be known for? Complaining or praising?

May you be known for living out your liberty in Christ with such joy and passion that other hearts see the way to lasting freedom and are changed from within.

ACTION STEP

Plan your workouts this week. Look at your schedule and write in the exact times you'll care for your body.

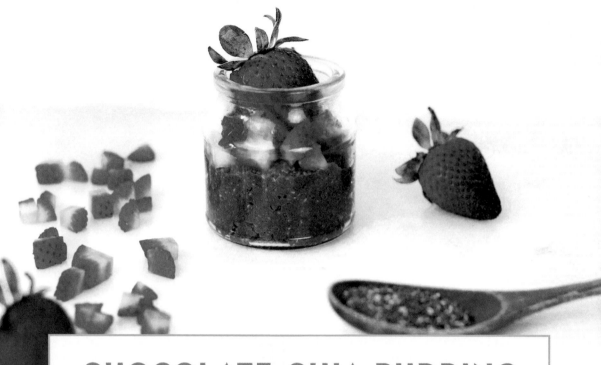

CHOCOLATE-CHIA PUDDING
WITH STRAWBERRIES

This tasty treat is sure to satisfy your sweet tooth! Chia pudding is filling and packed with healthy fats that are amazing for your brain and skin health. I love to whip this up in the morning and enjoy it later in the afternoon.

PREP TIME: 2–24 HOURS   YIELD: 1 SERVING

1½ cups almond milk
3 T. maple syrup
3 T. cacao powder

½ cup chia seeds
Fresh strawberries

Blend the almond milk, maple syrup, and cacao powder until fully combined. Stir in the chia seeds and let the mixture set in the fridge for a couple of hours or overnight. Top with freshly chopped strawberries and enjoy!

38

BRAVE
Today

THINK OF A TIME WHEN YOU SUMMONED THE COURAGE to do something, but as soon as you took the first step, fear crept into your heart. That has happened to me so many times. Fear of making the wrong choice. Fear of something terrible happening. Fear of messing up. Fear of not finishing. Fear of not making it. Fear here. Fear there. Fear everywhere.

Fears give power to insecurities that should not have a grip on us. We have no reason to fear when we're rooted in the love of God. First John 4:18 says, "There is no fear in love; but perfect love casts out fear, because fear involves torment. But he who fears has not been made perfect in love." When you allow the truth of who you are in Christ to change you from the inside out, you'll find the courage to move forward through security in God.

Take your fears to their rightful place, the feet
of Jesus. Leave them there and let love in.

I used to think that in order to move forward, fear needed to be absent, but Franklin D. Roosevelt was right in saying, "Courage is not the absence of fear."

Looking back over my life, I can testify that this is true. Fear was not absent when, as a 12-year-old, I was scared to leave home for camp, but I packed up my bags, faced the unknown, and ended up fully surrendering my life to Jesus Christ. There was my 18-year-old self's moment of panic when I decided to be unfettered by the popular opinion that college was the only next step, to trust God and do what I love and serve people. Then there was 21-year-old Cambria's leap of faith, the moment I decided I wasn't too young to marry my best friend and discovered the most wonderful gift in marriage.

FREE UP YOUR SPIRIT

God is with us despite our fear. I believe that God's Word so often says "do not fear" because it's something we do so often. But through the power of God's love, He gives us the courage to continue as He walks with us every step of the way, whether it's baby steps or leaps of faith. Take a moment to look back on your recent days:

- What are three ways you've been brave during this journey of health?
- What fear has God walked you through that used to prevent you from becoming strong in body and soul?
- Which baby step or nudge forward shifted you toward fitness progress this month?
- What is one fear you need to leave at the foot of the cross today?
- What keeps you moving toward the hope and future God has for you?

We are not abandoned in the fear-filled places of our lives. We will not be left alone on the wayside of our worried path. There is no need to panic or freeze up. We can free up our spirits instead. We can move ahead and transform fear with God-given courage to take one step at a time. Our greatest strength is found in the smallest of faith.

"If you have faith as a mustard seed, you will say to this mountain, 'Move from here to there,' and it will move; and nothing will be impossible for you."
MATTHEW 17:20

Keep moving forward in your purpose. Brave today with courage in Christ. Take your fears to their rightful place, the feet of Jesus. Leave them there and let love in.

ACTION STEP

Move more today. No big plan. No pressure. Simple.

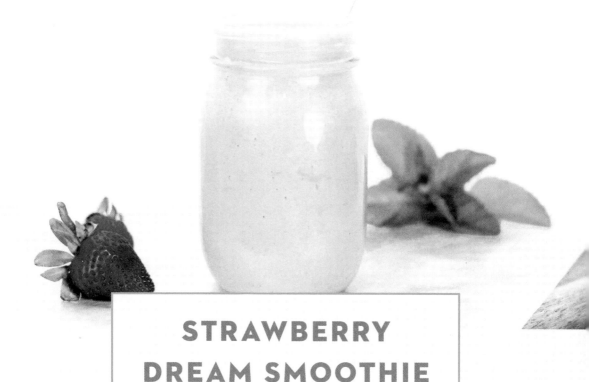

STRAWBERRY DREAM SMOOTHIE

This strawberry dream smoothie is exactly that—a dream. Light, refreshing, and completely heavenly, this smoothie packs a flavorful punch! It's healthy and simple, and I can't wait for your taste buds to try this and fall in love!

PREP TIME: 5 MINUTES   YIELD: 1 SERVING

3 large frozen strawberries
1 cup frozen pineapple
½ banana
splash of orange juice

splash of almond milk
(add until desired consistency)
honey to taste

Blend all ingredients in a blender until smooth.

39

THE
DANDELION
Wish

CLOSE YOUR EYES, MAKE A WISH, AND BLOW. That's what I used to do all the time as I held up dandelions and made wish after wish with great anticipation. You can make a wish any day of the year with these magical plants. The thing is, these little dreamy plants are weeds. They grow like wildfire. They're insidious. According to the Oxford Advanced Learner's Dictionary, "insidious" means "proceeding in a gradual, subtle way, but with harmful effects."

I remember when I made a particular wish. It was innocent; yet slowly but surely, I began experiencing its harmful effects. It was subtle. Gradual. All I wanted was to be happy. But I wasn't placing my hope in God. I was wishing on the lies of the world, and they seemed to multiply each time I closed my eyes and wished harder. The weeds of falsehood grew, spread, and soon were choking the life out of me and the garden God had created within me. Eating was no longer a joy because of my self-dictated restrictions and frequent guilt. Exercise wasn't fun; it was mandatory. Appreciating my body wasn't possible until I reached my unrealistic goal. This wish was turning into my worst nightmare, and it happened so inconspicuously that I had no idea.

Our desires can become the weeds in our internal garden, and they will keep growing if they are left to flourish. If we're not careful, they can choke the life out of every good thing.

TRANSFORMED BY THE GARDENER

Check out this verse: "The seed that fell among the thorns represents those who hear God's word, but all too quickly the message is crowded out by the worries of this life and the lure of wealth, so no fruit is produced" (Matthew 13:22 NLT). Did you catch that? "All too quickly..." It happened so fast—the good seed was crowded out by weeds and unable to grow. The truth of God's Word tells us that our worth is found not in our appearance but in Him. Our lives become beautiful when tended to by the Master Gardener. He clears the deceptive weeds, His Word enters our hearts and takes root, and our lives produce fruit of the spirit, not weeds.

I don't want to be choked out by the weeds, and I don't want you to be either.

Eating healthy is good but it's not the most important thing. Having good abs and a closet full of clothes might be blessings, but those are definitely not the important things. Matthew 6:25 (NIV) tells us, "Do not worry about your life, what you will eat or drink; or about your body, what you will wear. Is not life more than food, and the body more than clothes?"

When we abide in truth, we grow in truth. We can cultivate an abundance of joy that nourishes others rather than a scattering of seeds that will only take root to destroy someone else's garden.

Close your eyes, say a prayer, and grow with God.

ACTION STEP

Pray today about specific struggles you have when it comes to healthy eating and exercise, and write them in your prayer journal.

HIIT IT

LEVEL: CHALLENGING

TIME: 25 MINUTES WITH REST

ROUTINE: DO EACH EXERCISE FOR 45 SECONDS, RESTING 20 SECONDS BETWEEN EXERCISES, 5 SETS

Get ready to hit this high-intensity interval training workout (that's what HIIT stands for). Give it all you've got, and watch as you reach new limits in your fitness game.

▶ TURN TO PAGE 221 TO ACCESS VIDEOS FOR THIS WORKOUT!

PLANK JACKS

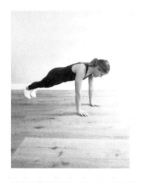 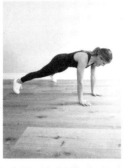 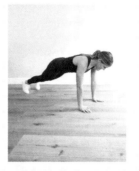 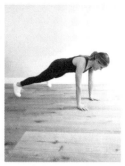

MOUNTAIN CLIMBERS

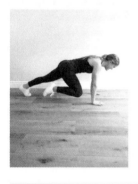 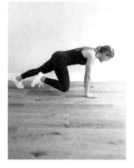 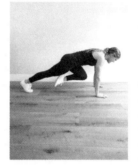 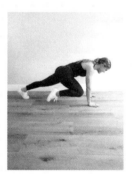

TOE REACHES

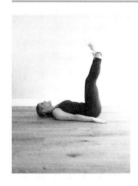 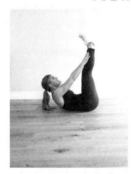 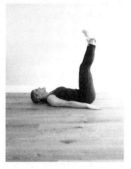 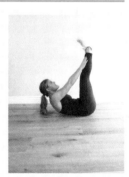

BURPEES TO TUCK JUMPS

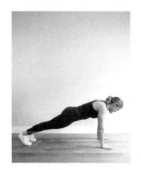 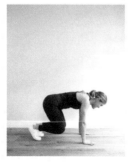 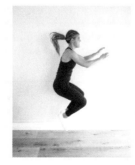 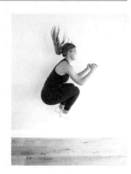

40

HEALTH
Food

BITE INTO THAT BACON BURGER, that spinach and strawberry salad with extra feta—oh, and the hot fudge sundae finale. Enjoy it. Savor it. Get crazy happy over it. We are free in Jesus to eat and enjoy food. I mean it. And I'm not going to list how many burpees you need to do to burn off the calories. Health food is the food that feeds your body and spirit. It doesn't bring you down or hurt you physically or spiritually. You know about moderation and balance. And in your transformation, you'll discover what works.

During a youth group trip to Yosemite, I experienced the freedom that comes with a healthy balance. Under the starry night sky, we gathered at the campfire to sing worship songs and eat s'mores. Normally I would have declined the gooey treats, but God had begun His deep work in my heart, so I reached for a couple and enjoyed every bite. As I wiped some graham cracker crumbs from my lips, I realized I was satisfied to stop at two. It was the strangest and best feeling.

After the fellowship time, my friend Ashley and I walked along a trail together. In the peace and stillness, I shared with her that God was doing a new thing in me. I confided how much weight I had gained from binge eating. I wasn't saying it out of

The good news is this:
Free will allows us to choose well.

shame, but because I knew God was glorified in my story. All of it. And I prayerfully, carefully share that with you now knowing that mention of weight gain can be triggering for some. I want to illuminate the gifts of this difficult journey. The early years were tough, but they were also the most healing and redemptive of my life.

Being honest with my friend was liberating. I told her I enjoyed the couple of s'mores that night without guilt or the compulsion to keep eating. We praised God for this new journey of true health. That night I felt full spiritually. A satisfying abundance in God is far better than the never-satisfied restriction of our bodies.

Colossians 2:16–17 says, "Let no one judge you in food or in drink, or regarding a festival or a new moon or sabbaths, which are a shadow of things to come, but the substance is of Christ." There are those today who still desire to judge you and me. Especially concerning healthy eating. And everyone thinks they're right. But here's the thing: Jesus had no patience for legalism. Jesus died to free us from the law and make us alive in Christ through grace and forgiveness despite what we do or even what we choose to eat.

First Corinthians 6:12 says, "All things are lawful for me, but all things are not helpful. All things are lawful for me, but I will not be brought under the power of any." Catch that? We are free to do what we want, but not everything we do will be good for us. Okay, we learn this early in life—probably in kindergarten, if not before. But somehow it doesn't sink in. We have to relearn the lesson that some things just aren't good for us. The good news is this: Free will allows us to choose well.

THE BUFFET IS OPEN

You are free to choose what you want to eat, and your health journey is your own personal story between you and a personal God! And your doctor. Medical and professional support and counsel will keep your choices safe.

Our attempts to help others with solutions, even with the best intentions, can sometimes turn into judgments if we are not careful, and that's why I never mention what you should or shouldn't eat throughout this book. That's not up to me, and I recognize that God has given us all the opportunity to choose.

Whatever we choose to do, we can give God thanks. We'll stay healthy longer if our decisions don't cause us to look down on others in judgment. What's also true is that we can enjoy our trip through the buffet line without anyone telling us what we should or shouldn't stack on our tray. The slice of apple pie stays, and the side of lies and guilt goes.

Let God guide you to health and healing. James 4:12 says, "There is one Lawgiver, who is able to save and to destroy. Who are you to judge another?" Just as there's not just one right way to exercise, there's not just one right way to eat. Your healthy life buffet is going to look different from mine.

You're free to take care of your body in a way that works for you.

ACTION STEP

Celebrate your freedom today by baking up a special treat!

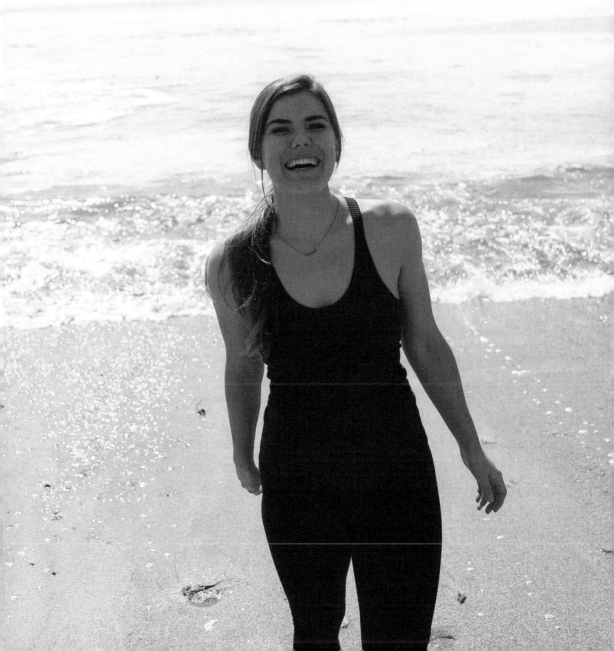

THE *slice of apple pie* STAYS,
THE *side of lies and guilt* GO.

41

TRADING GOOD FOR *Goodness*

MY LIFE IS FILLED WITH GOODNESS NOW. But it has taken time and wisdom and reliance on God to stand where I am today. There are still hardships. But the view from where I am now amazes me. I'm grateful that God guided me from a life of trying to be good to a life of grace drenched in His goodness.

When I initially turned my focus toward fitness, I did so for two main reasons: to prove to myself that I could win at this and to prove to others that I wasn't a failure.

Honestly, I thought my intentions were fine. They were driving me, that's for sure. The problem is, they were driving me in the wrong direction. I wanted to prove myself right and prove others wrong. Sure, I wanted to look good, but I also wanted to be good at all that I did.

I didn't have the spiritual eyes to see where that mentality was taking me. My energy was spent perfecting and performing. The goal ultimately was to please myself and

Trust that what God is doing in His grace surpasses the human version of good that you and I settle for in our day-to-day.

become the world's version of who I should be. That can often happen in life with our plans. We think we know the way, yet we end up at a dead end, thinking, "How in the world did I get here?"

CALLED BY GOD'S GOODNESS

Thank the Lord the growing process is redeeming. Even when we go in the wrong direction, thinking we are right, God uses our missteps not just to help us reach our final destination but also to change our hearts. Why? Because of grace—the one thing that changes everything. Grace covers our mess-ups, missteps, and mishaps.

What I thought I needed and what God knew I truly needed were two separate things. God's transformation in us starts in the heart. His grace reformed my desire to look and be good into a passion for knowing and trusting true goodness. He is doing that in you, too if you are growing in Him. First God calls us by His goodness, and then He invites us to add goodness to our faith so that we may continue to grow—not in perfection but in love.

His divine power has given us everything we need for a godly life through our knowledge of him who called us by his own glory and goodness. Through these he has given us his very great and precious promises, so that through them you may participate in the divine nature, having escaped the corruption in the world caused by evil desires.

For this very reason, make every effort to add to your faith goodness; and to good-
ness, knowledge; and to knowledge, self-control; and to self-control, persever-
ance; and to perseverance, godliness; and to godliness, mutual affection; and to
mutual affection, love. 2 PETER 1:3-7 NIV

Are your plans maybe not working out as you thought they would? Did you think
you were headed in the right direction only to end up wondering if you took the wrong
fork in the road? Maybe you just feel flat-out alone. Or maybe you reached your destination only to be disappointed.

There's a good chance that your intended destination isn't the one God has planned
for you. He will continue to shape you as you take steps in faith so you will be prepared for His plan. Trust that what God is doing in His grace surpasses the human
version of good that you and I settle for in our day-to-day.

Be encouraged. Turn toward joy in your health journey.

ACTION STEP

Pretend your reusable water bottle is a part of you and take it with you
everywhere you go. Whether you're sitting at your desk, running errands,
or at the gym, it goes where you go.

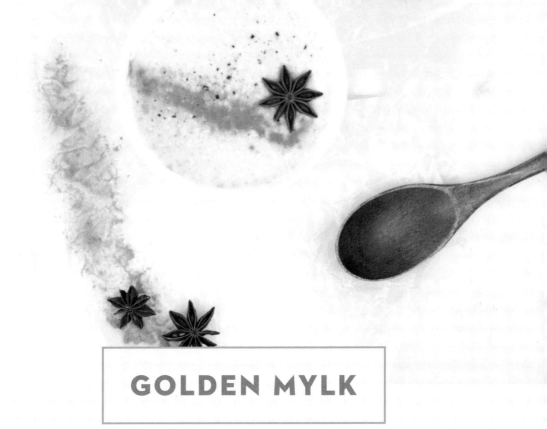

GOLDEN MYLK

This spicy, warm drink is an incredible anti-inflammatory that will bring a little zing into your life. A soothing mug of this beverage makes for an exceptional nighttime ritual. I sip on this before bed while reading a book.

PREP TIME: 10 MINUTES   YIELD: 1 SERVING

1 cup Homemade Almond Milk (page 25)
$\frac{1}{2}$ tsp. fresh ground turmeric
1 tsp. maple syrup
$\frac{1}{4}$ tsp. cinnamon

Pinch of cardamom
Pinch of ginger
Pinch of black pepper

Blend all the ingredients. Pour into a saucepan over low to medium heat to reach the desired temperature. Enjoy!

42

GOD PREVAILS
IN
Human Fails

DELIGHTING IN SCRIPTURE IS LIKE EATING A TOOTSIE POP:
You mull over a verse for so long, and then you finally get to the yummy center—the
aha moment. I had this experience the day I read of the apostle Paul's struggle with a
thorn in his flesh. The Bible doesn't say what that thorn was, but it may have been
a physical illness or a weakness. Paul pleaded and begged God to remove this thorn
from him. The Lord responded, "My grace is sufficient for you, for My strength is
made perfect in weakness" (2 Corinthians 12:9).

Hold everything!

The truth of this verse illuminated a falsehood I held tightly: My insufficiencies
are my identity. End of story.

Have you ever thought you were beyond hope because of your physical, human
failures? The truth is, our weaknesses make us more qualified to step into

> The degree to which you let go of control will be the degree to which you experience freedom in your soul.

God's grace and experience His strength: "For when I am weak, then I am strong" (2 Corinthians 12:10). When we are at our weakest, we are strong through Him. It's not that He gives us some superstrength. He Himself *is* our strength.

THE MYTH OF CONTROL

We think taking control means empowerment. What it means is that we take control out of the rightful hands of our loving Creator. He wants the best for us, and He knows what that is. We get antsy, agitated, or self-assured and start to tug parts of our life back from His possession. Then we wake up some Wednesday and realize our hopes have slipped through our fingers and we are surrounded by our handcrafted mess.

I encountered that truth when I desperately needed it. It was a day I thought I had my habits under control. It was a day that should have ended in physical victory. However, the control I thought I had was an illusion. By evening, I had negated my "successful" day of limited carbs with a binge of ice cream, bread, and cereal. Putting my hope in my own strength had left me burdened and a mess. Everything from my hunger to my emotions was more out of control than ever.

I reread the words of the Lord: "My strength is made perfect in weakness." My human frailty is an opportunity to lean into God's faithfulness and His sure strength. I glorify God not because I am perfect but because He is.

My pastor says that hope means the absolute expectation of coming good. I believed that if I followed my diet plan perfectly, the coming good would be a sense of satisfaction and worthiness. It was a case of misplaced hope. My expectation of coming good would be realized not through my efforts but in God. "You are my hope, O Lord God; You are my trust from my youth" (Psalm 71:5).

The coming good God has planned for us is so much better than our limited versions. When we give God, who is our hope, control over every area of our lives, we find the truth in Psalm 73:26: "My flesh and my heart fail; but God is the strength of my heart and my portion forever." Let God be the strength of your heart so that He will transform every human failure into eternal victory.

The degree to which you let go of control will be the degree to which you experience freedom in your soul. Transform weakness into strength...not in a lifetime of working out but in a moment of surrender.

ACTION STEP

Try a new type of exercise that you've never done. Sign up for a class and focus on enjoying new movements rather than checking it off your list.

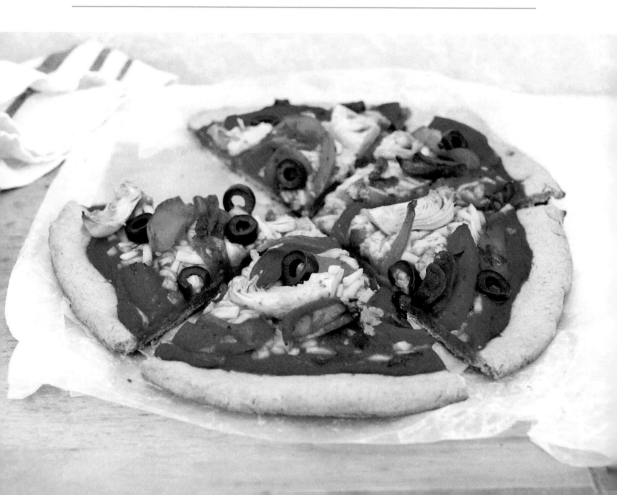

PANTRY PIZZA

This is one of my favorite go-to dinners. I usually whip up a gluten-free pizza crust (I like grain-free crusts or cauliflower crusts), but to keep things simple, you can grab a premade crust from the grocery store. I always buy premade organic pizza sauce and keep it in my pantry for ease. The point of this dinner is simple—to use what you have on hand. This is one of my favorite recipes of all time, and I have it at least once a week!

PREP TIME: **25 MINUTES**   YIELD: **4 SERVINGS**

---

1 red bell pepper, chopped
1 sweet onion, chopped
1 T. avocado oil
Pizza sauce
(enough to cover the crust to your liking)
Cooked vegetables of your choice
Premade pizza crust

Marinated artichokes
Olives
Garlic salt
¼ tsp. dried oregano
¼ tsp. dried basil
Salt and pepper to taste

Preheat your oven to 375°. Chop the bell peppers and onions, and sauté in avocado oil in a pan over medium heat until soft. Arrange the pizza sauce on top of your crust, and add cooked veggies on top. Finish by topping with artichokes and olives and sprinkling the garlic salt and spices on top. Add salt and pepper to taste. Bake for 10 minutes or until heated through.

43

HEART
Surgery

WHEN MY DAD HAD TO HAVE EMERGENCY open-heart surgery, I prayed that God would give him a phenomenal surgeon—one with a steady hand and many years of practice. A surgeon who had done this surgery plenty of times before. That was my first thought.

I *didn't* think, *This isn't just a matter of adding a few stitches; this is full-on open-heart, open-chest surgery. That's too deep of a cut. This is not happening, not on my watch; it's just too dangerous. Don't fix the diseased arteries!* I didn't go there mentally because as scared as I was, it would have been deadly to prevent a surgeon from making a new way for blood to flow in and through the compromised heart.

Just as my dad could not be made whole unless heart surgery was performed, the same is true for us, my friend. Our spiritual hearts need to be fixed. We feed ourselves lies, and soon they pool and gather and block our hearts. We need the Master Surgeon to cut in and reroute pathways so truth can flow in and out. When we surrender our hearts into the hands of this Master, there's no safer place to be. It's more dangerous to not have the surgery, because the Bible tells us, "Above all else, guard your heart, for everything you do flows from it" (Proverbs 4:23 NIV).

Sometimes God takes away
something to make us whole.

Here is the amazing thing: Sometimes God takes away something to make us whole. He removes the lies and idols in our hearts in a loving way so that our wholeness is found in Him alone. And the most gracious thing of all is that those scars from our pain don't remain; God turns them into beauty marks. They are eternal reminders of grace and transformation. What could be more beautiful?

Like a surgeon who creates incisions that are deep but healing, God does not allow needless pain. In Christ, our pain is never in vain. God can transform the very thing that brought us pain into what will ultimately bring us joy. Only a loving God would do that.

On a personal note, when I was caught in the spiral of binge eating, all I wanted was for God to take away the external manifestation of my behavior without the spiritual heart surgery. Sure, it would have been nice if a Band-Aid and gummy vitamins had been the cure, but this hurt, this need, was too deep.

I needed God to do what He lovingly does: correct me, chasten me, guide me, and eliminate anything that wasn't serving the King and His purpose for me—His daughter, His patient. God knows where to find our problems, our hurts, and our hang-ups. And remember, "Happy is the man whom God corrects; therefore do not despise the chastening of the Almighty. For He bruises, but He binds up; He wounds, but His hands make whole" (Job 5:17-18).

That's what God does for us. He makes a new way. He bruises and He wounds, but He binds us back up and His hands make us whole.

ACTION STEP

Do an arm workout today, and as you lift up the weight, think of it as handing your weights and needs to God.

READY, SET, SWEAT!

LEVEL: **MODERATE**

TIME: **25 MINUTES WITH REST**

ROUTINE: **DO EACH EXERCISE FOR 1 MINUTE, 3 SETS**

Don't think that you have to use a cardio machine to break a sweat!
This simple but effective workout will do the trick.
Get ready, get set . . . it's time to sweat!

▶ TURN TO PAGE 221 TO ACCESS VIDEOS FOR THIS WORKOUT!

JUMPING ROPE

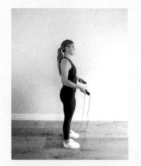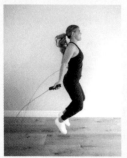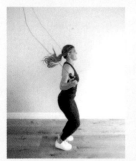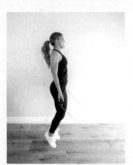

PLANK

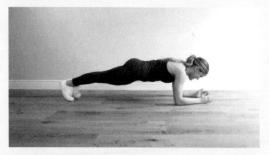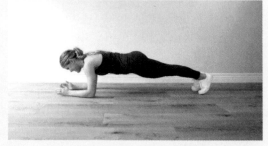

QUICK FEET

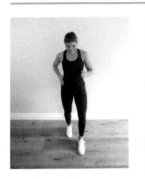 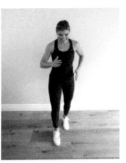 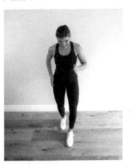 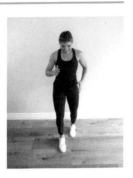

MOUNTAIN CLIMBERS

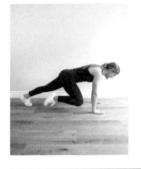 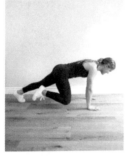 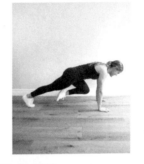 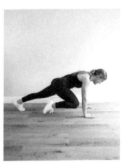

JUMPING JACKS

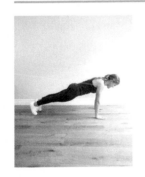 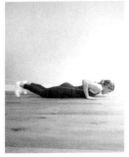 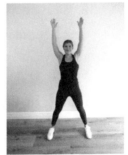 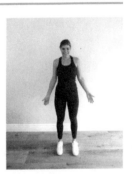

LAY-DOWN PUSH-UPS

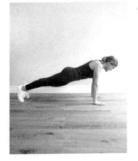 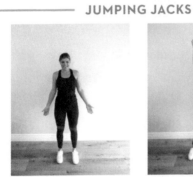 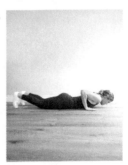

44

LAUGH
Today

A GOOD GAUGE OF PROGRESS AND CHANGE IS our response to circumstances—or potential circumstances, as may be the case.

There was a time when I wondered if I would ever live a healthy, balanced life. Anytime I made progress, I worried about whether I would fall back into old obsessions and patterns. Would an event or life hardship cause my trust in God's faithfulness to lessen? In hindsight, I realize that I worried about everything! I had grown, but I hadn't changed how I looked at the future or the possibility of failure.

Once I gained momentum making healthy decisions and healing choices, I started to examine the fear. There had to be a better way to go through life! I was starting to get energy from my workouts. Facing meals wasn't a trigger for spiral thinking anymore. I was ready to view today and tomorrow with hope.

In my reading of the Bible, I returned to Proverbs 31. I've heard it many times, so truthfully, it's a chapter of Scripture that I had been glossing or skipping over because I thought I knew what it had to share. But on this day, I felt led to spend time with it. I settled into a favorite chair with a cup of tea and let the words enter my heart in a way I hadn't before. "She is clothed with strength and dignity, and she laughs without fear of the future" (Proverbs 31:25 NLT).

The verse became a question, and I asked myself, *Do I ever laugh without fear of the future?*

I'd like to say yes, but that'd be a lie. I'm an excellent worrier, if I do say so myself. I can find just about anything to worry about. Especially my future. That's why I focused on and prayed this verse until I could grasp how to follow the example of the woman it describes. I realized that laughing without fear of the future is possible only if we give our worries to the One who holds that future: "[Cast] all your care upon Him, for He cares for you" (1 Peter 5:7). I hope you find these insights challenging in the best way. Lay your worries down at the feet of Jesus. We can be worry-free when we know our future is secure in God.

LAUGH TODAY, TRUST TOMORROW

Do you know who the author of Proverbs 31 is? While it isn't certain, there is speculation that Lemuel is Solomon. Proverbs 31 (KJV) starts off by saying, "The words of king Lemuel, the prophecy that his mother taught him." If in fact Lemuel is Solomon, that means the mother is Bathsheba. And who is she? She was the woman King David saw on the roof bathing. Long story short, King David committed adultery with her and got her pregnant. Her husband was then murdered, and her baby died. She was an adulteress, and her story has some other deep scars.

This woman had every reason to think that God wouldn't use her because of her mistakes or that circumstances would never get better because of the pain she endured. But guess what? God used this woman, who messed up and went through grief, to share with you and me how a virtuous, godly woman laughs without fear of the future.

Now *that's* security.

God holds your future, friend. Something beautiful is on the horizon, and that something is heaven. And between here and there is a path of truth and grace that blooms with blessings. Wherever you're at, no matter what you've done or what you're going through, lift your eyes to Jesus, who loves to fix what's broken and use it for something amazing.

Scripture flows with insight about the basics of life, including our tendency toward daily fear: "Therefore do not worry about tomorrow, for tomorrow will worry about its own things. Sufficient for the day is its own trouble" (Matthew 6:34). Jesus is very real with us. He isn't sugarcoating life when He acknowledges that today has enough trouble. A life of faith means we get to live fully in the moment. Fear of the future no longer has a hold on us. Sometimes that fear may creep in, but Jesus frees us from it if we let Him.

When we release worries about today, God changes our fear into joy for tomorrow. Don't let the enemy of tomorrow enter in the door of today. Look at what concentration camp survivor Corrie ten Boom said about that: "Worry does not empty tomorrow of its sorrow. It empties today of its strength." Isn't that the truth. Have you ever wasted a completely good day agonizing over something that might or might not happen a week later? We don't have to do that anymore.

God is the creator and ruler of time. He is just as much a part of tomorrow as He is of today. And of this moment. He is with you now. Just because you haven't made it to tomorrow doesn't change the fact that He's already there. Isn't that comforting? Empowering?

We are on a journey to become strong in spirit and body. Let's protect our todays. What is on your heart or your path today that you need help with?

ACTION STEP

Go for a prayer walk next time you feel worried, and leave your headphones at home. Walk and talk with God.

WE CAN BE *worry-free* WHEN WE KNOW OUR FUTURE IS *secure in God.*

A ONE-WEEK FOOD SAMPLER

What a journey, right? This has been an important time of seeking health and well-being within and without. To help you as you continue on your personal path, here is a one-week sampler of food, inspiration, and training to encourage your path. You know I don't like rules or rigid instructions. And this does not represent all the food you would have in a day by any means...because there should be more cupcakes! This is your foundation for each day to add to and build on. For more encouragement, check out my connection page so we can stay in touch and keep building each other up.

MONDAY

Food highlights: Grain-Free Granola (page 81) with Homemade Almond Milk (page 25) for breakfast, a salad with fruit for lunch, The BEST Peanut Butter Cookies (page 69) for a snack, and a favorite dinner of your choice.

Inspiration: Start with a prayer and journal time in the morning and before bed. Reflect on an inspirational verse.

Training: Set a date with a friend today to start walking together regularly. Start the week with fitness and fellowship!

TUESDAY

Food highlights: Over-easy eggs with a side of avocado and fruit for breakfast, a Simple Nourish Bowl (page 61) for lunch, a Blueberry Milkshake (page 37) for a snack, and a new dinner to keep it fun.

Inspiration: As soon as you wake up, read your Bible for 10 minutes. Keep it by your bed and read a psalm to start your day.

Training: Lower-Body Toner workout (page 208) and a 20-minute low-intensity steady-state walk.

WEDNESDAY

Food highlights: Smoothie of choice for breakfast, Immunity-Boost Chicken Soup (page 101) for lunch, Gorilla Milk (page 105) with a handful of nuts and a piece of fruit for a snack, and Pantry Pizza (page 191) for dinner.

Inspiration: Write down your food and workout choices today and record how you feel. This isn't about calorie counting or restricting. This exercise is about becoming more in tune with your body and recognizing what foods and workouts energize you. Keep track for a week and then look back to see how you felt. Do you recognize a pattern?

Training: Full-Body Sculpt workout (page 136).

THURSDAY

Food highlights: Acai Bowl (page 155) for breakfast, a tuna salad with avocado and lemon dressing for lunch, Iced Matcha Latte (page 125) and Stuffed Medjool Dates (page 132) as a snack, and for dinner, a Grain-Free Tortilla (page 133) stuffed with a favorite cooked protein and grilled veggies and topped with salsa or guacamole.

Inspiration: Try a heart-rate monitor in today's workout. See if you can push yourself to maintain 80 percent of your maximum heart rate during your workout.

Training: Ready, Set, Sweat! workout (page 194).

FRIDAY

Food Highlights: Breakfast Quinoa (page 145), a Simple Nourish Bowl (page 61) for lunch, Chocolate-Chia Pudding with Strawberries (page 171) for a snack, and Sheet-Pan Fajitas (page 163) for dinner.

Inspiration: Find a way instead of an excuse. On your crazy-busy days, getting in a ten-minute workout at home is a positive day. Thank God for your ability to move.

Training: Abs on Fire workout (page 212).

SATURDAY

Food highlights: Poached eggs over roasted sweet potato with side of spinach for breakfast, tomato soup and a garden salad for lunch, a Strawberry Dream Smoothie (page 175) for a snack, roasted veggies over quinoa with tahini dressing for dinner, and grain-free homemade cookies for dessert.

Inspiration: Swap a store-bought treat for a homemade treat. Get creative in the kitchen and try to make your favorite pre-packaged treat at home with wholesome ingredients.

Training: I Got Your Back! workout (page 52).

SUNDAY

Food highlights: Hard-boiled eggs with a banana and almond butter for an on-the-go breakfast, leftover paleo shepherd's pie for lunch, a banana and peanut butter smoothie for a snack, and for dinner, Hawaiian grilled skewers with chicken, bell peppers, and pineapple drizzled with coconut aminos.

Inspiration: Turn off social media today and spend time with God and your family. Have quiet time before bed. Write in your prayer journal as you pray over the upcoming week.

Training: Rest today. Use the foam roller to ease muscle tension, and take an Epsom salt bath.

45

LET GOD
Weigh In

YOU HAVE THE FINGERPRINT OF GOD ON YOU. You are made in His image according to His likeness. You can look in the mirror and say, "I am handmade by God, and my joy is found in my identity in Christ."

But do you do that? Do I do that? Not always. I've had long seasons when I looked to the scale to tell me what my image was and what it was worth. What happens, though, when we ask God to weigh in on our value? Read the following verse a couple of times, and let it be your morning-time meditation, or your workout focal verse, or all of the above! "A person may think their own ways are right, but the LORD weighs the heart" (Proverbs 21:2 NIV).

This Scripture stunned me. Back when I was stepping on the scale daily, sometimes multiple times, I was desperately trying to lose weight to gain value. I thought my way of measuring was right, but the Lord "weighs the heart." God measures what is going on inside us and what we treasure.

This truth leads us right back to ideas from the motivation section: God sees the inside. Our internal life of heart and spirit and mind matters more than the external life the world measures to indicate our success, worthiness, acceptability, likeability.

God weighs your heart.
You will never be a number to Him.

God weighs your heart. You will never be a number to Him. Spend time with God's Word to understand what God sees and knows about you so this can be your measure, your truth.

You are made in God's image.

So God created man in His own image; in the image of God He created him; male and female He created them. GENESIS 1:27

You are redeemed.

"Fear not, for I have redeemed you; I have called you by your name; you are Mine." ISAIAH 43:1

You are a child of God.

See what kind of love the Father has given to us, that we should be called children of God; and so we are. 1 JOHN 3:1 ESV

Blessed. Chosen. Holy without blame. Adopted. Accepted.

Blessed be the God and Father of our Lord Jesus Christ, who has blessed us with every spiritual blessing in the heavenly places in Christ, just as He chose us in Him before the foundation of the world, that we should be holy and without blame before Him in love, having predestined us to adoption as sons by Jesus Christ to Himself, according to the good pleasure of His will, to the praise of the glory of His grace, by which He made us accepted in the Beloved. EPHESIANS 1:3-6

Sink into the truth and let it do its transformative work in you. Release yourself from the burden of using weight or body type to provide you with something that only God can give you: satisfaction and value. With Jesus, you start at the finish line. God's Word has the final and only say, and it says you are beautifully and wonderfully made in the image of God.

We glorify God when we recognize that we are not our own. When we are transformed, He weighs our hearts and knows that our intentions are to praise Him. We are His daughters, created to please God, not ourselves. True joy is found when we lay ourselves down. The funny thing is, when we ask God to empty us of ourselves and be filled with Him, we will find we are fuller, more satisfied. We are also lighter, unburdened by false measures and voices.

You will be more motivated and delighted when planning your week of food, inspiration, and training the day you let God weigh in on who you are in Him. Your pursuits to be fit and healthy will pour forth from a transformed heart of gratitude.

ACTION STEP

Write a prayer on a sticky note today about what you specifically want God to help you with concerning exercise.

GOD ISN'T LOOKING FOR

THE ONE WHO GETS TO THE GYM EVERY DAY.

HE'S NOT LOOKING FOR

THE PERFECTLY HEALTHY EATER.

HE'S NOT LOOKING FOR

THE STRONGEST PERSON.

HE'S LOOKING FOR YOU.

Come to Him as you are.

46

A BEAUTIFUL
Balance

BALANCE AND MODERATION ADD sweetness, stability, and wisdom to our experience. What if we only ever read the book of Leviticus? We'd never understand the grace of God pertaining to our sin. But what if we only ever read the book of Galatians? We might feel free to walk in sin by abusing God's grace. That's why we have a balance of grace and conviction in the Bible. We need both. And a healthy diet requires balance. What if you only ever ate vegetables? If you never ate any fruit or had any protein, you probably wouldn't feel very well. That's why we eat a variety of different foods.

One of my favorite things about the Bible is that it answers our biggest and hardest questions and sometimes even our silly and small questions, reminding us that God cares for the details of our lives. Let's look at what Jesus says in Mark 7:18–19: "Do you not perceive that whatever enters a man from outside cannot defile him, because it does not enter his heart but his stomach, and is eliminated, *thus* purifying all foods?"

Cookies can't defile us, but our obsession with a perfect body can. Look at the next three verses:

The God who created the leaves in the salad we eat is the same God who created cocoa beans.

And He said, "What comes out of a man, that defiles a man. For from within, out of the heart of men, proceed evil thoughts, adulteries, fornications, murders, thefts, covetousness, wickedness, deceit, lewdness, an evil eye, blasphemy, pride, foolishness. All these evil things come from within and defile a man." MARK 7:20-23

It's not what goes into us that defiles us; it's what comes out of our hearts. How does this apply practically to our lives? Well, your body is the temple of the Holy Spirit. What's going on in your heart matters more than what's on your plate.

Eating healthy does not mean shunning chocolate forever. Unfortunately, I used to think it did. When I stopped dieting and started listening to my internal signals, God guided and helped me eat in a way that honored the body He gave me. For example, I knew that excessive chocolate or excessive sugar is not healthy. Proverbs 25:27 says, "It is not good to eat much honey; so to seek one's own glory is not glory." But depriving yourself of any and all chocolate forever isn't healthy either.

Back to balance.

May we take comfort in knowing that the God who created the leaves in the salad we eat is the same God who created the cocoa beans that make chocolate. By the grace of God, we'll live with balance and beauty. Bon appétit!

ACTION STEP

Ask yourself what you need the most out of your exercise routine right now. Fast, effective workouts? Slow, de-stressing movements? Maybe long runs for some me-time? Assess where you're at in your life, and fit your workouts to meet your needs.

LOWER-BODY TONER

LEVEL: **EASY**

TIME: **15 TO 20 MINUTES**

ROUTINE: **DO EACH EXERCISE FOR 1 MINUTE, 4 SETS**

Grab your mat and workout bands, and get ready to get in an amazing at-home workout!

▶ TURN TO PAGE 221 TO ACCESS VIDEOS FOR THIS WORKOUT!

BANDED SQUATS

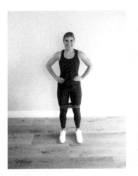 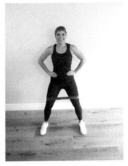 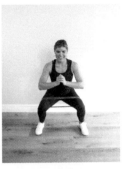 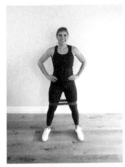

ABDUCTOR TAP OUTS

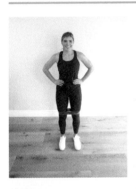 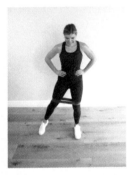 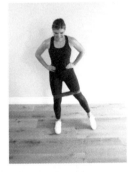 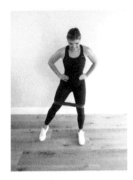

SQUAT JUMPS

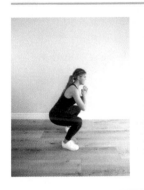 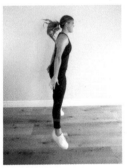 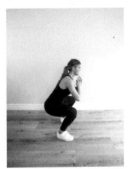 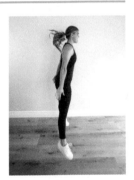

BANDED GLUTE BRIDGES

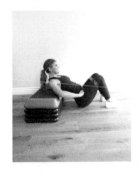 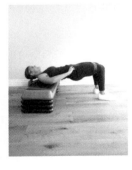 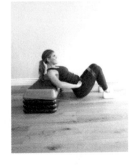 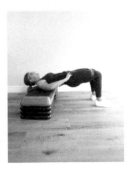

47

REAL

Progress

HOW IS IT GOING? How are you doing?

It's inspiring to look at the adventure we've embarked on together and how far along you are in your journey toward becoming fit body and soul. Take a quick glance back. Think about the day you started this book, and then consider how you feel about your physical and spiritual life today. Taking stock can be of considerable value as encouragement and as a path toward gratitude. Don't do it to judge areas that are lacking, but instead, spend this time acknowledging how far you have come—or rather, how far God has brought you.

PROGRESS BY GRACE

May you have the mind of Christ to know that your progress is not marked by perfection but by grace: "Grow in the grace and knowledge of our Lord and Savior Jesus Christ" (2 Peter 3:18). With that awareness, explore this list and sit with it. Embracing these truths is a measure of your growth in the knowledge of the Lord. Celebrate where you are in God's mercy:

My joy comes from the Lord and not from circumstances or the approval of others.

- I am loved by God.
- I am wonderfully made.
- My identity is in Christ alone. Nothing and no one else measures my worth or value.
- When I move and nourish my body, I do it to take care of what God has entrusted to me.
- I am physically stronger and spiritually able to lean into God's strength.
- My freedom is already secured in Christ.
- I can count trials and challenges as joys because God uses them to make me steadfast.
- God will fight for me.
- My joy comes from the Lord and not from circumstances or the approval of others.
- I am never apart from God. He is never apart from me.
- God has gone ahead of me and has a plan for my life.

Now it's time to move forward. Remember what Paul said in Philippians 3:13: "One thing *I do*, forgetting those things which are behind and reaching forward to those things which are ahead."

There is goodness and joy, hope and continued transformation on the path ahead. Thank God specifically for the progress that He's helped you with this far, and ask Him to help you keep your eyes on Him as you take the next step.

ACTION STEP

Write down your favorite promise from this list and read it throughout the day.

ABS ON FIRE

LEVEL: MODERATE

TIME: 18 MINUTES WITH REST

ROUTINE: DO EACH EXERCISE FOR 30 SECONDS, MINIMAL REST BETWEEN MOVES, 5 SETS

This workout will bring the heat...to your abs, that is! This quick ab challenge is perfect for tightening your core when you're running low on time. It packs a punch, so get ready to be sore! No equipment is required, so it's perfect if you're on the go.

▶ TURN TO PAGE 221 TO ACCESS VIDEOS FOR THIS WORKOUT!

PLANK

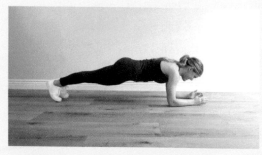 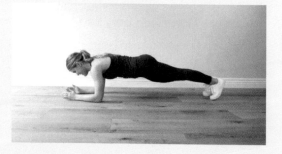

SIDE PLANKS

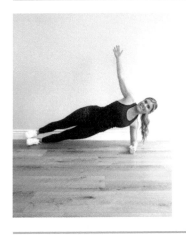 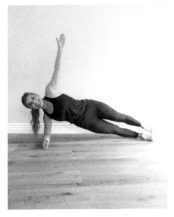 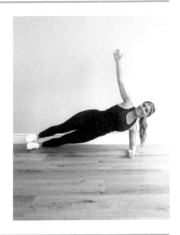

CRUNCHES

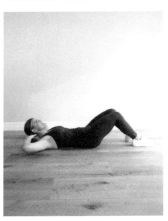 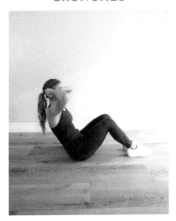 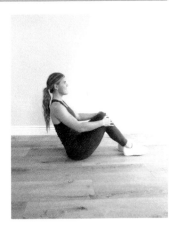

RUSSIAN TWISTS

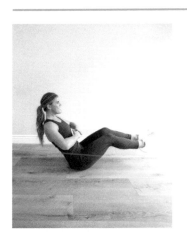 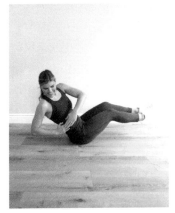 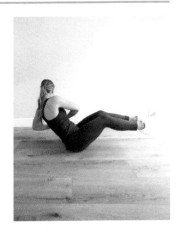

48

A HEART FIT
for Joy

AS YOU LOOK BACK OVER THIS JOURNEY we've had together, can you see how God has given you a heart fit for joy? What has changed in your daily walk with God and pursuit of health and wholeness?

When I get up in the morning, I feel the fullness of joy. God's joy. Even on days when I know I'll have a stretch of tough hours or a difficult situation that I'd rather avoid, I can push the covers aside and stand firm on the foundation of my hope and feel strong in my body and soul.

On days when old struggles or stumbles come to mind first, the grace that allows me to forgive my past is the grace that moves me—and you—into the future. Every day I depend on God's strength and grace for real change. The kind of change that allows me to live as His child and to live out my purpose with His joy at my core.

"These things I have spoken to you, that My joy may remain in you, and that your joy may be full" (John 15:11). Fullness…satisfaction. All from Him.

> A heart that is satisfied in
> God has no room for comparison.

A CHANGED HEART

As you feed and strengthen your spirit, your desire to reflect Jesus will fill your soul in a way you never thought possible. What the mirror shows doesn't matter on a soul-level anymore. What other people think about you doesn't rock you the way it used to. You will even find rest in your imperfections. Remember, God isn't looking for the one who gets to the gym every day. He's not looking for the perfectly healthy eater. He's not looking for the strongest person. He's looking for you. Come to Him as you are.

You're already perfect in His eyes. What Jesus did for us on the cross changes us within—we are holy and blameless. Ask God to transform your heart into a heart that is after His. A kingdom-seeking heart is a heart fit for joy. A heart that desires to know God above all else is a heart fit for joy. This heart helps you see yourself and the women around you through the lens of Christ: holy, adopted, blameless, perfect, beautiful, wonderfully made, handcrafted, and unique.

Rejoice today that He sees you and He has saved you! You are beautiful because He says so. Deuteronomy 7:6 says, "For you are a holy people to the LORD your God; the LORD your God has chosen you to be a people for Himself, a special treasure above all the peoples on the face of the earth." A special treasure. That's you! And what a delight to know the One who has never spoken anything but truth has spoken words of beauty over you.

ACTION STEP

Pray that God will help you take one step toward extending grace to yourself.

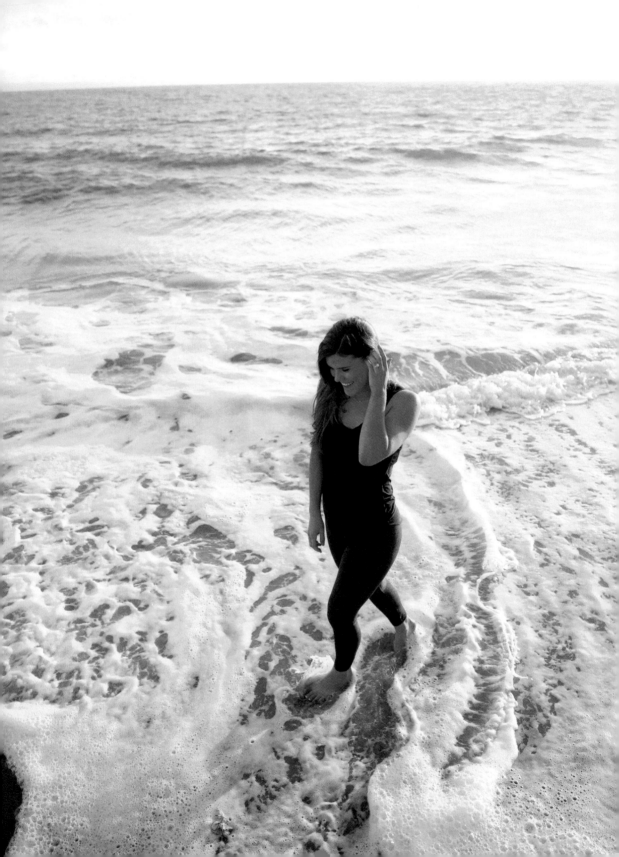

BE TRANSFORMED

We also glory in tribulations, knowing that tribulation produces perseverance; and perseverance, character; and character, hope.

ROMANS 5:3-4

I am sure of this, that he who began a good work in you will bring it to completion at the day of Jesus Christ.

PHILIPPIANS 1:6 ESV

We do not lose heart. Even though our outward man is perishing, yet the inward man is being renewed day by day.

2 CORINTHIANS 4:16

Even youths grow tired and weary, and young men stumble and fall; but those who hope in the LORD will renew their strength. They will soar on wings like eagles; they will run and not grow weary, they will walk and not be faint.

ISAIAH 40:30-31 NIV

Create in me a clean heart, O God, and renew a steadfast spirit within me . . . Restore to me the joy of Your salvation, and uphold me by Your generous Spirit.

PSALM 51:10, 12

Thank You for changing and perfecting me from the inside out, Lord. I'm so grateful for the chance to become strong and healthy physically. I pray to face each day with joy and an eagerness to walk boldly in the purpose You have for me. Help me taste and see that You are good so that even challenges lead me to rest in Your strength and glorify You. In Jesus's name, amen.

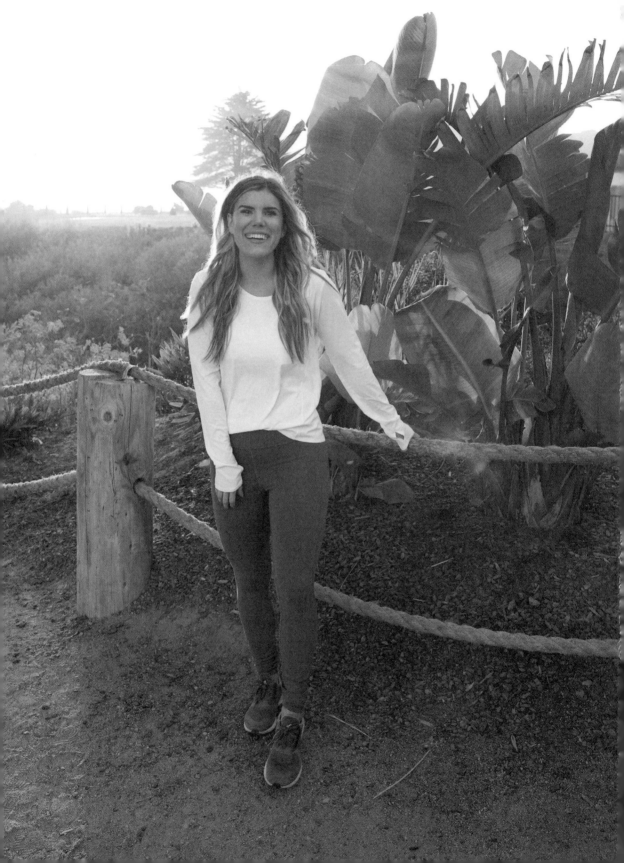

A NOTE FROM
Cambria

WE'RE HERE, AT THE END OF OUR TIME TOGETHER—at least through this book. I hope you'll find me online and tell me how you're doing. Before I go, I want to share some special words with you. There are three words that will save you a lot of heartbreaks and backaches. These three words can change the course of your story:

God is able.

When you surrender your transformation process to the Lord, God leads your body, mind, and spirit toward amazing inside-out changes and blessings. The new you is given a new view. That's what the gospel does for us—it presents the only reliable foundation of self-evaluation through the perfect mirror of the Word of God.

Your personal path of spiritual and physical health continues. So does mine. We can come back to these pages for a refresh, but our steps forward are with God and in His able strength. I wave goodbye and send you along with prayers for health and joy and the truth of three more words that you can hold on to with hope:

God is faithful.

My friend, God is faithful in all circumstances and at all times. He hears your prayers, and He loves you with an everlasting love. May you draw close to Jesus and desire to know Him and walk with Him all the days of your life. May your deepest desire be not to perfect your image but to reflect His image.

From my heart to yours,

Cambria Joy

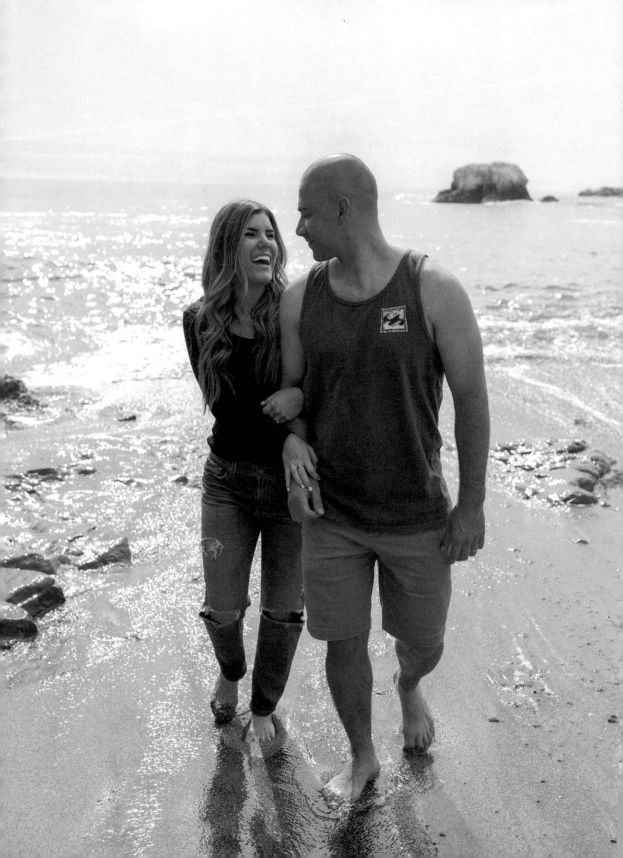

CONNECT WITH *Cambria*

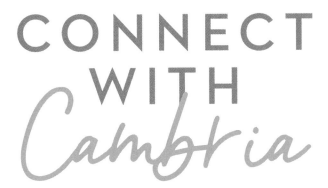

LET'S CONTINUE THIS STORY TOGETHER. You are so important to me. I can't wait to hear how you've grown in strength as you come to the end of this book and continue your journey. There are beautiful things on the horizon for you, my friend! I want to stay in touch.

For inspiring emails full of healthy tips and soul encouragement, sign up and join the community for free at CAMBRIAJOY.COM/SIGNUP

Watch my YouTube videos for a look into my life, my advice for you, workouts, recipe ideas, and lifestyle tips: YOUTUBE.COM/USER/CAMBRIAJOY

We can hang out daily on Instagram. I see this as my live journal, with personal thoughts and daily life moments: @CAMBRIAJOY

I hope you will return to the pages of this book and these social media outlets every step on your way to become motivated, strong, and transformed. I look forward to our ongoing adventure.

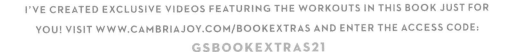

I'VE CREATED EXCLUSIVE VIDEOS FEATURING THE WORKOUTS IN THIS BOOK JUST FOR YOU! VISIT WWW.CAMBRIAJOY.COM/BOOKEXTRAS AND ENTER THE ACCESS CODE: GSBOOKEXTRAS21

INDEX OF
Recipes
and Workouts

EXERCISES

Cover design by Faceout Studio, Lindy Martin
Interior design by Faceout Studio, Paul Nielsen
Photography by Bo Dam-Mikkelsen

Growing Strong
Copyright © 2021 by Cambria Joy Howard
Published by Harvest House Publishers
Eugene, Oregon 97408
www.harvesthousepublishers.com
ISBN 978-0-7369-7806-4 (pbk)
ISBN 978-0-7369-7807-1 (eBook)

Library of Congress Cataloging-in-Publication Control Number: 2020027346

Printed in the United States of America

20 21 22 23 24 25 26 27 28 / VP-FO / 10 9 8 7 6 5 4 3 2 1